'If you or someone that you love is impacted by MS this book is a must read. The seven-step process for self-management presented in the *Overcoming Multiple Sclerosis Handbook* is a comprehensive and thoughtful approach to living your best life despite having this disease.'
Dr Aaron Boster, The Boster Center for Multiple Sclerosis, Columbus, Ohio

'This highly recommended book highlights the importance of a holistic approach to MS management, offering a path to achieve the best possible outcome in this potentially devastating condition.'
Professor Richard Nicholas, Imperial College London

'A deeply insightful account and instructive guide for adopting healthy lifestyle behaviors and thriving while living with MS.'
Dr Sarah Mulukutla, Founding Chairperson of the Section on Neurohealth and Integrative Neurology at the American Academy of Neurology, New York

'Written specifically for people who have MS, this inspirational book provides a comprehensive, practicable program for living a full life with this disease.'
Dr Alessandra Solari, Fondazione IRCCS Istituto Neurologico Carlo Besta, Italy

'Overcoming MS is now the essential mainstay of MS management, before or alongside drug therapy, offering the best chance of a full and healthy life for people with MS.'
Dr Peter Silbert, Clinical Professor of Neurology, University of Western Australia Medical School

'A wonderful resource for people living with MS.'
Dr Ilana Katz Sand, Associate Professor of Neurology, Icahn School of Medicine at Mount Sinai, New York

Overcoming Multiple Sclerosis Handbook

ROADMAP TO GOOD HEALTH

Edited by George Jelinek MD
Sandra Neate FACEM and
Michelle O'Donoghue MD MPH

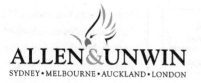

ALLEN&UNWIN
SYDNEY·MELBOURNE·AUCKLAND·LONDON

First published in 2022

Allen & Unwin
83 Alexander Street
Crows Nest NSW 2065
Australia
Phone: (61 2) 8425 0100
Email: info@allenandunwin.com
Web: www.allenandunwin.com

 A catalogue record for this
book is available from the
NATIONAL
LIBRARY   National Library of Australia
OF AUSTRALIA

ISBN 978 1 76087 878 8

Internal design by Midland Typesetters, Australia
Set in 11/15 pt Sabon by Midland Typesetters, Australia
Printed and bound in Australia by Griffin Press, part of Ovato

10 9 8 7 6 5 4 3 2 1

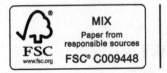 The paper in this book is FSC® certified.
FSC® promotes environmentally responsible,
socially beneficial and economically viable
management of the world's forests.

For Eva and Iva
—George Jelinek

For my brother, Colin
—Sandra Neate

To my family, in particular my husband Andrew,
for their unwavering support
—Michelle O'Donoghue

Contents

Foreword

The Overcoming Multiple Sclerosis 7 Step Recovery Program ('the OMS Program' and 'the Program') outlined in this book has the potential to radically change your life for the better. I know because it has changed mine. Even more importantly, nearly every contributor telling their story in the following pages is a testament to the power of the OMS Program too.

I first met Professor George Jelinek in 2002 in Melbourne, Australia, where he had just started running workshops for people with multiple sclerosis (MS). I was the 28-year-old woman slumped on a bright yellow beanbag in the middle of the room, struggling to get through each day, debilitated by an array of symptoms. Four months earlier I had received the devastating diagnosis, which explained the sudden and dramatic onset of symptoms that had engulfed my body and in turn my mind and spirit. It transformed me from a strong independent woman in the prime of my life to a bedridden shell of myself, reliant on others for care.

I sat among a room full of people, all there for a glimmer of hope from a man who himself had been dealt the same diagnosis and had witnessed his mother's decline and eventual suicide as a result of the same illness that had ravaged her body years earlier. At the time Professor Jelinek was considered somewhat of a revolutionary, some would even say a maverick. He had consolidated the evidence from around the world and put together a holistic lifestyle program that he believed had the potential to completely change the lives of people with MS.

For me it was a pivotal moment. As I embraced the OMS Program, it empowered me little by little to take back control of my health. It provided me with the evidence to understand why the recommendations work and it motivated me to do whatever it took to overcome MS.

In the subsequent years Professor Jelinek paved the way as a leader in the field, ultimately setting up, and then conducting health and lifestyle research in MS at, the Neuroepidemiology Unit (NEU) at the prestigious University of Melbourne.

When I set up the Overcoming Multiple Sclerosis (OMS) charity in the United Kingdom in 2012, it was with a passionate belief that this lifestyle information needed to be made available to every single person newly diagnosed with MS. I felt a sense of responsibility to share George's work, as I had experienced its life-changing outcomes at first hand. In fact, it felt negligent not to spread the word. If I could turn my health around, so could others; they just needed to be given the opportunity to understand the evidence underpinning the recommended changes.

And now, a decade later, the real testament to George's work is that this latest book is a handbook that is written by our community and for our community. It builds on his ground-breaking book *Overcoming Multiple Sclerosis: The evidence-based 7 Step Recovery Program*, which provides the detailed scientific evidence base of how changing one's lifestyle can positively affect the development and progression of MS.

Joining Professor Jelinek in bringing this book to fruition are two other editors from opposite sides of the world, steeped in medical and scientific expertise. Dr Sandra Neate is a specialist emergency physician who heads the NEU at the University of Melbourne but also has significant involvement in forensic aspects of medicine, in particular through the Coroners Court of Victoria and the Mental Health Tribunal in Victoria. She has also run many residential OMS retreats with George. With her academic rigour, Sandra bridges the divide between teaching and research in medicine and her practical clinical contributions, as well as her insider perspective on living for twenty years with someone who has lived and breathed the OMS Program.

Professor Michelle O'Donoghue is a US cardiologist and Associate Professor of Medicine at Harvard Medical School whom George and I met on the OMS tour of the United States in 2016 and who herself was diagnosed with MS in 2010. As a researcher and clinical trialist, she has a particular appreciation for the evidence on which the OMS Program is based.

These editors now release, for the first time, expanded practical information condensed into a simple, practical guide on how to follow the OMS Program, written so that anyone who has been touched by this life-changing condition can benefit. Nearly all the contributors, as well as being international experts in their own fields, follow the Program, having been diagnosed with MS themselves. They say that the job of a master is to create new masters and so it is hugely inspiring to read what these new masters of the OMS philosophy, from all corners of the world, have to say as they come together to share their insights. As you dive into this book, you'll find a manual brimming with super accessible, practical tools and information drawn from professional knowledge and personal experience.

Of course, the hard truth is that getting well from a diagnosis of MS is not plain sailing. Overcoming MS can be a long and hard road. The challenge is to remember that the setbacks and frustrations can lead to greater resilience, if we allow them. I remember the first day when taking a breath wasn't painful—it was a near miracle. And I also remember the days when a green hue overwhelmed my vision accompanied by inexplicable fatigue drowning my body after doing 'too much' the day before. I called them 'green days'.

But I maintained hope, which in time became faith and finally belief that the tools now presented in this book would help me to navigate the good days, the terrible days and everything in between. Slowly, over time my symptoms gradually improved until they completely disappeared, and I have been relapse-free ever since and no longer have any lesions detectable on MRI.

Research on diet and lifestyle is at the heart of the OMS Program, but on another level so is the wider offering of 'community'. We are naturally social beings, but ill health can be debilitating, isolating and lonely; it certainly was for me at times. Thankfully, the Program is a gateway to a community that quite simply understands what you are going through and that brings a shared sense of empowerment and belonging. For anyone recently diagnosed with MS, rest assured that the Program will connect you to a network of people enthused with realistic positivity and hope. You will not feel alone.

However, the Program has an even broader and more subtle contribution than just assisting those diagnosed with MS. It is a valuable tool for the families and loved ones who are also on this journey, offering practical approaches to how we can all live happier, healthier lives. After all, the true gift is in enabling the best not only for ourselves but also for those around us.

The good news is that there is a gradual turning tide of understanding about the benefits of a holistic approach to MS that works alongside conventional treatment. Though this awareness has been prominent in other chronic health conditions such as diabetes, heart conditions and cancer for some time, we are now seeing more people reporting that their neurologists are taking an interest. We are observing increasing cases of remission and of NEDA (No Evidence of Disease Activity) and we are hearing about neurologists looking for something more to offer their patients in addition to the pharmaceutical options. The change may be slow, but it is happening and as such this book has the potential to accelerate a paradigm shift in MS management globally.

Overall, this book's contribution to people with MS, their families and the wider MS community is extraordinary. I urge you to read it, absorb it, weave it into your own story, and share it with your family and loved ones. Through thick and thin, let this book become your trusted healing companion. It will empower you to live your best life. It has mine.

Linda Bloom
President
Overcoming Multiple Sclerosis charity
Buckinghamshire, United Kingdom

Preface

It sometimes astounds me that the one-page memo, stuck to the fridge at home, that I put together in 1999 to help me live well after a diagnosis of MS, has been of help to so many people around the world. Scientists globally have increasingly focused on researching this critically important area, with more and better publications accumulating, not least from some of the editors of and contributors to this book, validating the potential benefits of this risk-modification program. What else has happened, though, is that people who have adopted this way of living have added their own dimension and nuance to the prescription. This book is about those people, the Overcoming Multiple Sclerosis (OMS) community, the people whose lives have been touched by the OMS Program and who have agreed to share their insights and tried-and-true methods of adopting this lifestyle approach and living a full life.

I express my gratitude to all of the contributors, most of whom have MS diagnoses: those who have written comprehensive content chapters outlining a clear path for people adopting the OMS Program to follow; those who have penned their personal stories to illustrate how life has unfolded for them after embracing the Program; and those who have provided inspirational quotes to further personalise each of the chapters. This book is now truly representative of a wide section of the OMS community, not only lighting the way for other people with MS and their families to follow, but inspiring us with the affected individuals' strength, courage and determination. Research counts for a lot in medicine, but so does the lived experience of these trailblazers in showing us what a profound difference taking control of MS can make, that overcoming this disease can now be a reality for many, many people with MS.

Professor George Jelinek

~

The concept for this book began during a trip to the United Kingdom when the Overcoming Multiple Sclerosis (OMS) charity wondered how the ideas and suggestions in Professor Jelinek's book *Overcoming Multiple Sclerosis: The evidence-based 7 step recovery program* (1st edition, 2010, 2nd edition, 2016) could be made future-proof. Future-proofing involved writing a book that was less reliant on citing medical literature and more representative of the experience of people with MS. We also wanted to explore topics not previously covered in other MS texts, such as progressive MS, the role of families, work, disclosure, and pregnancy and the perinatal period.

As this idea of a multi-authored book written (largely) by people with MS who were actively engaged with modifying their lifestyles developed and we approached people with invitations to write chapters and provide their personal stories, it became apparent that there was a vast wealth of knowledge and experience in the OMS community that had been untapped. The concept of a book written by the OMS community for the community of people with MS continued to evolve, and this is the end product.

I come from a background of emergency medicine, a frantic-paced specialty of medicine where we deal with the end product of illness and injury. Working over many years now with people with MS, and being a part of the team at the Neuroepidemiology Unit at the University of Melbourne where we research lifestyle modification in MS, I have experienced great joy in working with people in a collegial manner, forming lifelong relationships with them, being a part of a shared experience and striving towards health improvement and, hopefully, prevention.

I have enjoyed watching the chapters and stories contained therein unfold. Each chapter author has drawn from their expertise in the area, but also from their own unique experiences and perspectives. They bring insights into the barriers and challenges they have faced and their own very personal and, what were until now, private ways of facing those challenges. They have shown remarkable courage in sharing their experiences. These sentiments apply equally to the other individuals who have contributed personal stories within each chapter. I hope our book provides not only detailed information but also insights and inspirations from this remarkable group of people to assist you whether you have been diagnosed with MS or, like me, are sharing your life with someone diagnosed with MS.

Dr Sandra Neate

~

I will never forget the moment when the neuro-ophthalmologist turned his back to me and announced to a group of medical students, 'As you can see, this patient's brain MRI has all the classic findings of multiple sclerosis'. At that moment, I felt like the rug was being pulled out from under me and I broke down sobbing. Those words changed my life forever.

It was only a few days earlier that I had begun to lose vision in my right eye when I was returning from a medical conference. Over the course of two days, my vision loss rapidly progressed until I was completely blind in that eye. As a physician, the possibility that my symptoms could be explained by MS had entered my mind, but I had promptly dismissed it. 'How could I have MS?', I had asked myself. With those words, I shifted into a phase of several months of denial as I moved through the stages of grief.

Fortunately, the possibility that diet and lifestyle may play a role in the progression of MS immediately felt right to me. If the body was inappropriately attacking itself, it seemed probable that something was driving that confusion and that I might be able to play a role in altering its course. During my first meeting with the neurologist, I asked him about the role that diet might play and he told me that some people believed in the work of Dr Roy Swank. I read Dr Swank's book and soon thereafter came across the book *Overcoming Multiple Sclerosis* by Professor Jelinek.

As a physician, I appreciated the fact that Professor Jelinek had researched the field extensively and presented his recommendations based on the best available evidence. Nonetheless, I will fully admit that when I first read his book, I was not yet ready to hear his message or embrace the necessary changes. Instead, I followed the path of more traditional medicine and started daily injections that were quickly upgraded to intravenous medication as my MRI showed further signs of progression. My scans revealed that I had more than 25 brain lesions and several appeared to be new. During this time, I had convinced myself that the dietary changes recommended by Professor Jelinek were just too challenging, and I seemed to relish going out to restaurants to eat soft cheeses and meat with my friends as my disease continued to progress.

I can't tell you exactly when something shifted inside me. After several months, I went back to my bookcase and re-read Professor Jelinek's book. The next day, I woke up and adopted all of his recommendations. It's now been a little more than ten years since my diagnosis and I'm delighted to report that I have yet to suffer a single clinical relapse and my brain MRI has remained stable. Although I am eternally grateful for my physical health, I am even more appreciative of the lessons that the OMS Program has taught me about myself during this unexpected journey.

Above all else, George's OMS Program delivers hope and inspiration to people with MS at a time in their lives when things may seem quite hopeless. The first books I read following my diagnosis all painted a bleak picture of an inevitable downhill decline. Professor Jelinek gave me back a sense of optimism and a sense of control over a disease that terrified me. In turn, the OMS Program has also made me a better physician as I have gained a deeper understanding of the role that diet and lifestyle may play in so many different disease processes. In that sense, I truly believe that one has nothing to lose by embracing Professor Jelinek's recommendations, as these changes can only lead you to a place of enhanced physical and spiritual health.

When George approached me to help him co-edit this book, I was grateful to have the opportunity to help promote his message of optimism for people with MS. For those of you who have already embraced the OMS Program, I hope that this book helps to reignite your commitment. For those of you who may have struggled or not yet embarked on this path for self-improvement, I encourage you to keep an open mind and allow yourself to be inspired by the possibility that you may have more control over your fate than you previously realised. There is reason to see light on the horizon and remain optimistic!

Associate Professor Michelle O'Donoghue

About the editors

Professor George A. Jelinek MD, MBBS, DipDHM, FACEM

George Jelinek is one of Australasia's pioneer emergency physicians, having served as President of the Australasian Society for Emergency Medicine, Vice-President of the Australasian College for Emergency Medicine, the first professor of emergency medicine in Australasia and Founding Editor of the journal *Emergency Medicine Australasia*. After his diagnosis with MS in 1999, he devised the OMS Program, and founded and headed for its first three years the Neuroepidemiology Unit at the University of Melbourne. He has devoted his life to bringing a message of hope, optimism and good health to people with MS everywhere. He has twice been a state finalist for Australian of the Year for his contribution to MS and emergency medicine.

Dr Sandra L. Neate MBBS, DRANZCOG, DA(UK), GradCertForensMed, FACEM

Sandra Neate is a medical professional of 35 years' experience, having trained and worked in a variety of service, teaching and research roles as a specialist emergency physician, including as Medical Director of Organ Donation at St Vincent's Hospital Melbourne. She has had considerable experience in the forensic aspects of medicine, including a decade investigating deaths in healthcare facilities for the Victorian State Coroner, and sitting on the Mental Health Tribunal in Victoria. She has published extensively on emergency medicine, organ donation and MS. Sandra now heads the Neuroepidemiology Unit at the University of Melbourne.

Associate Professor Michelle O'Donoghue MD, MPH

Michelle O'Donoghue is Associate Professor of Medicine at Harvard Medical School and a practising physician and cardiologist at Brigham and Women's Hospital in Boston. She earned her medical degree from Columbia University College of Physicians and Surgeons in New York City. She subsequently completed a Master of Public Health at the Harvard School of Public Health. She has been involved in many international randomised controlled trials and published extensively in high impact medical journals. Michelle was diagnosed with MS in 2010 and adopted the OMS lifestyle shortly thereafter. She has lived free from clinical relapses since that time.

About the contributors

Dr Brandon Beaber is a neurologist and MS specialist in the Southern California Permanente Medical Group. He is the author of several publications on MS epidemiology and has participated in clinical trials for MS therapeutics. He makes YouTube videos about MS and posts about MS news and research on Twitter as @Brandon_Beaber. He lives in Los Angeles with his wife and two children.

Dr Virginia Billson graduated with a Bachelor of Medicine and Bachelor of Surgery (MBBS) degree from the University of Melbourne in 1973, then specialised in pathology. She worked as a specialist histopathologist at the Repatriation General, Royal Melbourne, Mercy and Royal Women's hospitals; at the latter, she was Director of Anatomical Pathology from 1995 to 1999. She was diagnosed with RRMS ('relapsing remitting MS') in 1996 and remains well by following the OMS philosophy.

Dr Annette Carruthers AM is a general practitioner (primary care physician) in Lake Macquarie in New South Wales and a Conjoint Senior Lecturer in the School of Medicine and Public Health at the University of Newcastle. She fulfils several roles on different boards involving financial services, health, infrastructure and aged care. She is a past president of MS Australia. Annette adopted the OMS Program in 2001. Dr Carruthers was awarded a Member of the Order of Australia (AM) in 2021 for her services to people with MS.

Dr Sam Gartland is a general practitioner in northern New South Wales and facilitates OMS retreats. Sam was diagnosed with MS in 2008; he has now recovered by following the OMS Program.

Associate Professor Craig Hassed OAM is coordinator of mindfulness programs across Monash University. He was the founding president of Meditation Australia, is a regular media commentator and has published thirteen books. He has co-authored the world's two top-ranked free online mindfulness courses. In 2019 Craig was awarded the Medal of the Order of Australia (OAM) for services to medicine.

Greg Hendron is a 46-year-old lawyer living in Northern Ireland with his wife Caroline and his two small children Darragh and Ronan. He was diagnosed with MS in May 2010 and adopted the OMS Program in June 2010. Greg has been and continues to be integral to the growth of the OMS community in Northern Ireland.

Rebecca Hoover earned a Bachelor of Science in Business degree from the Carlson School of Management at the University of Minnesota where she also studied in MBA and PhD programs. She has worked as a finance and information technology manager and consultant in small to medium-sized international organisations. She is now a vice president at a law firm focused on social justice. Diagnosed with MS in 1991, Rebecca adopted the Swank MS diet in the late 1990s and the OMS Program in 2007.

Dr Rachael Hunter is a mother of two, a chartered clinical psychologist and Senior Lecturer in Clinical Psychology at Swansea University in Wales. Diagnosed with MS in 2012, Rachael adopted the OMS Program straight away.

Dr Pia Jelinek graduated in medicine from Notre Dame University in Fremantle in 2016. After four years of hospital medicine, she is now practising family medicine in Perth. Pia has published five papers on MS prevention, contributed to facilitating OMS retreats in Australia and has a long experience of living with a devotee of the OMS Program, her father George.

Dr Conor Kerley was diagnosed with MS at the age of fifteen after three major relapses in nine months. Inspired by his circumstances, Conor became a Doctor of Nutrition, working at universities and health centres in Ireland and the United States. Published in international peer-reviewed medical journals, his research includes twelve papers on the role of vitamin D in the treatment of MS. Eighteen years after diagnosis, Conor is symptom-free, relapse-free and medication-free.

Dr Heather King is a general practitioner in Auckland, New Zealand. She is an OMS retreat participant, partner, mother, GP, equestrian, gardener and lover of life in general. Heather adopted the OMS Program in 2004.

Karen Law is a singer/songwriter and guitar teacher from the Sunshine Coast, Queensland, who adopted the OMS lifestyle after her diagnosis in 2010. A former journalist, she co-wrote the book *Recovering from Multiple Sclerosis: Real life stories of hope and inspiration* with George Jelinek and has carried out several volunteer roles within the OMS charity. She is married to David and together they have three children.

Jack McNulty has been involved in food and cooking most of his life. He has worked for chefs in high-end restaurants in Switzerland, Italy and France, and operated his own catering business and cooking school. He has provided recipes and information to the OMS website and was the contributing editor to the *Overcoming Multiple Sclerosis Cookbook*. Jack has followed the OMS lifestyle since 2009.

Dr Phil Startin, after obtaining a doctorate in physics, worked for Price Waterhouse as a management consultant for over 20 years. Since 2014, Phil has delivered the Mindfulness Based Stress Reduction (MBSR) course. He is a facilitator for the OMS charity, a trustee at MS-UK, and is currently working on a variation of the MBSR course specifically for people with MS. Phil was diagnosed with primary progressive MS in 2007, adopted the OMS Program in 2012, and attended the first OMS retreat in the United Kingdom in 2013.

Dr Keryn Taylor is a psychiatrist with clinical experience in neuropsychiatry, psycho-oncology and perinatal psychiatry. She is an Honorary Senior Clinical Research Fellow at the Neuroepidemiology Unit, University of Melbourne, and is an OMS retreat facilitator. Diagnosed with MS in 2005, Keryn adopted the OMS Program the same year. She remains well.

Dr Jonathan White is a UK obstetrician and gynaecologist, with interests in early pregnancy and recurrent pregnancy loss. He assists the OMS charity as a medical adviser and event facilitator. He lives and works on the north coast of Northern Ireland, sharing his life with his wife and two young sons, and enjoys the great outdoors, cycling, rugby, reading and film. He adopted the OMS Program the week after his MS diagnosis in 2015.

Dr Stuart White continues to work full-time as a consultant anaesthetist in Brighton, United Kingdom. He has published numerous research papers on a variety of subjects, including medical law and ethics, hip fracture management, and the environment. He was diagnosed with MS aged 40 in 2010, and has enthusiastically followed the OMS Program since 2016.

Part 1
The lay of the land

1

Understanding multiple sclerosis

Dr Brandon Beaber

Seek help and find your own personal path through what seems like a wilderness; but it's not, there are bluebells to be found in the fog.

Christine Nolan, Belmont, Australia, OMSer

She has a confident look as though her time might be better spent outside my office. The tingling in her left arm barely lasted a week and didn't impede a single spin class or Zoom meeting. She's twenty-four, fit, worldly and ambitious—the owner/operator of a search engine optimisation consulting business. She's been everywhere, knows people in high places, and you couldn't guess her ethnicity after five tries. She boasts coiled hair professionally dyed with blond streaks, a Louis Vuitton handbag, and clothes that must cost more than my entire wardrobe. She is the paragon of millennial money, both street and book smart with the right balance of entrepreneurial risk-taking spirit and seventy-hour-a-week discipline.

Onyeka (her name and some details of her life have been changed for privacy) shifts her countenance when I show her the MRI scans (Figures 1.1, 1.2).

She queries: 'How could a symptom so brief and trivial look terrifying? Is that really my MRI? What is this mysterious illness, and what will happen to me?'

Multiple sclerosis (MS) may invoke negative imagery for some of those unfamiliar with the disease: they think of wheelchairs and nursing homes. But Onyeka is typical of the patients I see. The trouble with MS is the fear and uncertainty about the future it causes. Though I desperately want to, I can't give her a prediction of what course her MS will take, a timeline or a guarantee. Onyeka is not the type to wallow in despair, and she hits me with

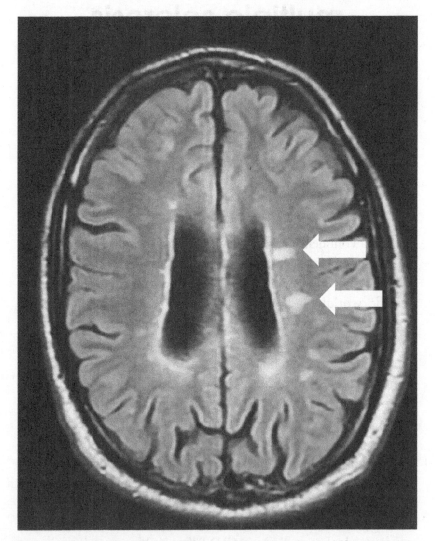

Figure 1.1: An axial T2 FLAIR MRI scan of Onyeka's brain. MS lesions are the small white areas flagged with arrows.

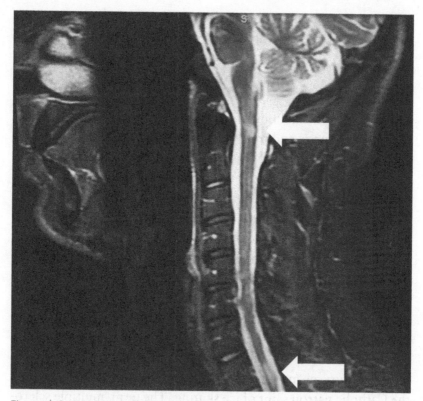

Figure 1.2: A sagittal T2 STIR MRI scan of Onyeka's cervical spine. The MS lesions are flagged with arrows.

a laundry list of questions and an interrogating tone I might resent if the circumstances were different. She is looking for what psychologists call the 'internal locus of control' and wants to know what she can do to better her situation. Given you are reading this, I suspect you have a similar mindset.

Some time ago, I set out to read every book about lifestyle and MS, determined to best them all by researching and writing my own manuscript. It was to be inspired by science rather than anecdotes, more up-to-date and evidence-based than anything before. However, when I read *Overcoming Multiple Sclerosis* by Professor Jelinek, I concluded I had been beaten to the punch, and as far as I can tell, his recommendations reflect the best available evidence, so I am following the old idiom: 'If you can't beat 'em, join 'em'. I am honoured to introduce the roadmap provided by this handbook to help you face MS with courage, conviction and wisdom.

What is MS?

The purpose of this book is to put into context the role of lifestyle in the genesis and treatment of MS, but we must begin with a foundation of general knowledge. MS is an interesting and complex disease, so consider this a brief overview and framework for future chapters. The disease is believed to affect over 25,000 Australians,[1] nearly one million Americans[2] and several million people worldwide. The lifetime risk of MS in developed countries with high prevalence is about one in 350 or ~0.3 per cent, which has been rising significantly in recent decades.

MS was first formally described by the French neurologist Jean-Martin Charcot in 1868, and the last century and a half has brought some understanding to this mysterious illness, the first recording of whose symptoms may have been as early as the fourteenth century, as manifested in Lidwina the Virgin (1380–1433), the Catholic patron saint of ice skating. The term 'multiple sclerosis' refers to hardened (or 'sclerotic') scars (plaques) in the brain, optic nerves and spinal cord. When we look under the microscope during a biopsy or autopsy, we primarily see damage to the myelin, a fatty sheath that protects nerve fibres (Figure 1.3).

The nervous system is essentially the organ of communication within the body, so when myelin is injured by what is currently thought to be an autoimmune process (i.e., when the immune system attacks our own bodily tissues), the speed and integrity of information transmission along nerves are hindered. This gives rise to the myriad symptoms MS can cause: vision loss, numbness, weakness, imbalance, tremor, problems with bladder and sexual function, pain, fatigue, vertigo, double vision, cognitive changes, and so forth.

MRI scans are helpful for diagnosis and monitoring of MS because they allow us to see lesions (the visible areas of damaged nerves) in a living person. MS lesions appear bright on what is

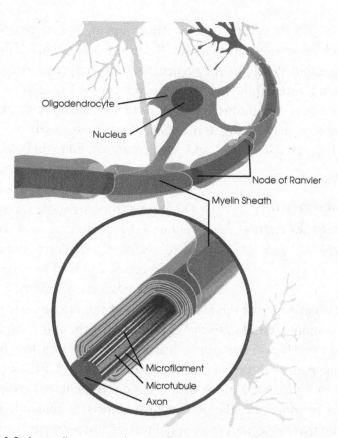

Oligodendrocyte

Nucleus

Node of Ranvier

Myelin Sheath

Microfilament

Microtubule

Axon

Figure 1.3: A myelin-covered nerve fibre is like an electrical wire with insulation. Oligodendrocytes are cells that produce myelin in the central nervous system. Source: Wikimedia Commons.

termed the T2 sequences of the MRI scan, and with permanent nerve fibre loss, they may be dark on T1 sequences ('black holes'). An active lesion causes a temporary breakdown of the blood-brain-barrier (the normal membrane separating the brain from the blood), and gadolinium contrast dye given before the scan can seep into the lesion, causing it to 'enhance' (appear brighter). Partly as a result of this damage, the brain can atrophy (shrink) in MS by a rate of ~0.5–1.35 per cent per year.[3] We monitor MS with routine exams and periodic MRI scans because new MS lesions often develop in the absence of symptoms.

New MS symptoms usually show up in one of two ways: through relapses or progression. Relapsing MS is marked by relatively rapid development of neurological symptoms over days to weeks, often followed by improvement and quiescence. We call the new symptoms 'relapses' and the intervening periods are 'remissions'. Many terms are synonymous with 'relapse', including 'attack', 'flare' and 'exacerbation'. Sometimes attacks are mild, such as slight numbness of the left hand that resolves in a week. Other times they are more severe and followed by prolonged and incomplete recovery. On rare occasions a single attack can lead to major permanent irreversible disability.

The severity of MS attacks varies greatly

As an example of the manifestations of the disease, one of the most common initial signs of MS is optic neuritis, or inflammation of the optic nerve. Symptoms usually include vision loss in one eye and pain with eye movement. It preferentially affects colour vision and the centre of the field of vision. If the initial visual loss is mild or moderate, the outcome (prognosis) is generally good, with improvement occurring spontaneously or after oral or intravenous steroid treatment.

In contrast to relapsing MS, progressive MS is slow and insidious, with an absence of the clearer episodes of neurological impairment that define relapsing MS. Symptoms gradually worsen over many months or years, and we often recognise the onset retrospectively after significant changes have accumulated. Gait and mobility are commonly affected, but some people may experience progressive imbalance, cognitive decline or any other symptom caused by MS. For unknown reasons, progressive visual loss is rare.

What are MS subtypes?

For most people, MS starts in the relapsing phase ('relapsing remitting MS' [RRMS]) without obvious progression. Some with RRMS will later in the course of the disease develop steady downhill progression, with or without relapses, known as a transition to 'secondary progressive MS' [SPMS]. About 15 per cent of people with MS start off with progressive disease, known as 'primary progressive MS' [PPMS]. Figure 1.4 (A, B, C) shows a representation of possible disability changes over time for the three main MS subtypes referred to here.

Younger people are more likely to have relapsing MS, and older people are more likely to have progressive MS. Some with progressive MS also have relapses, and, importantly, there is robust evidence that people with relapsing MS often have subtle unrecognised progression.[4] Irreversible disability in MS is primarily driven by progressive disease rather than relapses. There is strong epidemiologic, imaging, genetic and pathological evidence that all forms of MS share a similar underlying pathological process, so the three subtypes are useful mostly as descriptors and do not indicate truly distinct diseases.

Is there a test for MS?

Unfortunately, there is no single definitive test for MS. The diagnosis is usually based on a history of symptoms, a physical exam and MRI scans showing lesions typical of the disease. Sometimes additional testing can help confirm the diagnosis. For instance, blood tests can be helpful to rule out diseases that mimic MS, such as vitamin B12 deficiency, Lyme disease or other autoimmune diseases. Although less common in modern times, a procedure called a spinal tap, or lumbar puncture, can be useful. For this test a needle is introduced into the lower back under local anaesthesia to draw out cerebrospinal fluid (CSF) that surrounds and supports the spinal cord and brain. About 90 per cent of people with MS have abnormal antibodies in the CSF that are not in the blood. After a laboratory procedure called gel electrophoresis, these antibodies show up as bands of dark pigment called 'oligoclonal bands'.

To look for signs of old optic nerve injury, a test called 'visual evoked potentials' can be helpful. For this study, electrodes are placed on the back of the scalp, and a special checkerboard pattern of light is flashed into the eyes. The speed of transmission through the optic nerve can be measured, revealing signs of subtle damage.

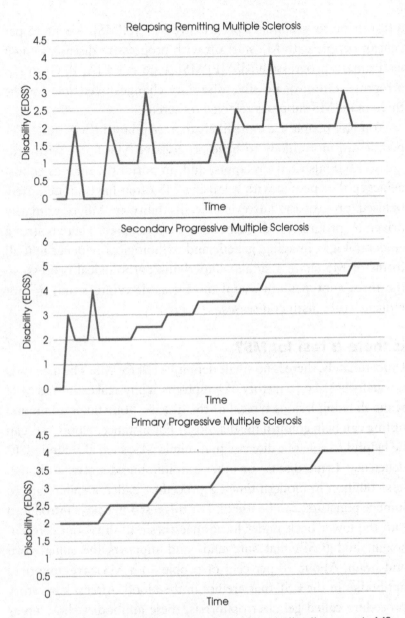

Figure 1.4 (A, B, C): Disability changes over time in the three main MS subtypes. Time is shown on the horizontal X-axis, and a measure of disability called the Expanded Disability Status Score (EDSS) is shown on the vertical Y Axis. EDSS is a discrete scale where values can only be whole or half numbers up to 10, but in progressive MS, changes are often smooth and continuous rather than discrete. Note that disability typically accumulates over time with all types of MS.

Taken together, the symptoms, physical exam and test results can help to support or refute a diagnosis of MS.

There are also formal criteria for diagnosing MS, most recently formulated as the 2017 revised McDonald criteria. However, MS can be difficult to diagnose accurately because many symptoms may be caused by myriad other conditions, and lesions showing in MRI scans can be benign or caused by other diseases. Hence, MS is very commonly misdiagnosed, and I am often 'undiagnosing' people with MS, even in situations where they have carried the diagnosis for years and received numerous treatments. If there is any doubt, you may consider a second opinion.

MS is commonly misdiagnosed

How bad is MS?

One thing that always strikes me is how dramatically the severity of MS varies from person to person. This is one of the most typical features of the disease. For some people, it is possible to see MS plaques at autopsy despite no history of symptoms during life.[5] Others have mild MS with good recovery from relapses and live long lives despite no specific treatment. Still others have varying degrees of moderate problems from MS, perhaps doing well for decades but acquiring disabilities later in life. An unlucky few have rapidly progressive MS or even a fatal disease course. It may frustrate the reader to learn that I ask every single person I meet with so-called benign MS how they manage their condition, and very few of them follow a particularly strict diet or lifestyle. Individual randomness is part of the mystery of the disease.

No guru, regardless of experience or professional qualification, can give any meaningful prognosis to someone with MS. There is simply too much variability. However, we can get a sense of the average rate of progression by looking at groups of people with MS over time. These studies usually use a measure of disability called the Expanded Disability Status Score (EDSS), which is commonly used in MS research and clinical trials (Table 1.1), although some self-reported measures of disability are also used.

Drawing from the MS-EPIC study from the University of California San Francisco,[6] of those who start with relapsing MS, the proportion who require a cane to walk 100 metres (EDSS 6.0) is 4.7 per cent at 10 years, 16.2 per cent at 20 years, but over 50 per cent at 40 years. The rate of transition to secondary progressive MS is 6.4 per cent at 10 years, 24.2 per cent at 20 years, but over 50 per cent at 40 years. But while the average age of diagnosis is thirty, and many will therefore have problems later in life, these statistics are for all people

In clinical trials, MS disability is usually measured with the Expanded Disability Status Scale (EDSS)

Table 1.1: The Expanded Disability Status Scale (EDSS)

EDSS	Description
0	No disability
1.0–2.0	Minimal disability
3.0–4.0	Moderate disability
4.5	Can walk 300 m
5.0	Can walk 200 m
5.5	Can walk 100 m
6.0	Cane needed to walk 100 m
6.5	Walker required to walk 20 m
7.0	Wheelchair required. Cannot walk more than 5 m
7.5	Wheelchair required but can walk a few steps
8.0	Unable to stand up
8.5	Mostly restricted to bed. Some use of the arms
9.0	No use of the limbs. Able to speak and eat
9.5	No use of the limbs. Cannot speak or eat
10	Death due to MS

Note: The scoring under the EDSS is complex and requires a neurological examination, so I have simplified the information in this table.

with MS, and we don't yet have good data on how adopting the OMS Program will affect this.

Furthermore, those with progressive MS at the onset are more likely to have significant disability at diagnosis and have a much worse prognosis on average. That being said, we think MS is becoming milder over time. The numbers above look good compared with older natural history studies, which revealed a nearly double risk of cane use after 25 years.[7] The probability of reaching EDSS 3, 4 and 6 is decreasing in Sweden.[8] This may be due to the use of disease-modifying medications, vitamin D supplementation, or higher rates of diagnosis in people early in the course of MS or with milder disease who may not have been diagnosed in the past.

The MS-EPIC study found that after twenty years people with relapsing remitting MS (RRMS) have a 1 in 6 chance of needing a cane and a 1 in 4 chance of transitioning to secondary progressive MS (SPMS)

Many believe that the EDSS scale is too focused on walking ability and misses the subtler symptoms of MS. Overall, 40–65 per cent of people with MS have objective signs of cognitive impairment, meaning difficulties with memory, perception or judgement on formal neuropsychiatric testing,[9] and these may not be obvious to a casual observer. Demyelination (loss of myelin) in regions connecting disparate areas of the brain influences processing speed and multitasking ability. For example, I have a patient who is a highly intelligent accountant but cannot meet the demands of fourteen-hour days during tax season. Indeed, many will rate invisible symptoms such as fatigue, pain and cognitive 'fogging' as their most severe symptoms. MS symptoms may be overt and covert.

What causes MS?

The medical consensus is that MS is an immune-mediated disease where white blood cells invade the central nervous system, similar to how the immune system attacks joints in rheumatoid arthritis. These white blood cells are effectively 'confused', and target the person's own proteins instead of foreign viruses and bacteria, causing inflammation of that part of the nervous system. Myelin proteins are a major target of these unhinged defenders.[10] This is why the term autoimmunity is used to describe the process. There is also evidence of degeneration in MS such as failure of mitochondria, the energy-producing machines within the cells. Researchers have found 'smouldering' inflammation in old MS plaques invisible to conventional MRI scans.[11] Over time, 'naked' nerve fibres without their myelin protection may fail.[12]

Part of the risk of developing MS is simply genetic—that is, the information that determines certain biological characteristics is passed from parents to offspring. Relatives of people with MS have a higher risk of developing the disease, and the stronger the genetic relationship, the greater the risk. I compiled an approximate risk of different types of relatives from multiple sources in Table 1.2. MS is not transmitted from parent to child by individual genes like in cystic fibrosis or polycystic kidney disease. Rather, numerous genes each contribute a tiny proportion of risk or protection. Almost all of these genes have something to do with the immune system, coding for cell-surface proteins on immune cells or cytokines, the chemicals involved in immune signalling. The gene most associated with MS is HLA DRB1*1501, which is part of the major histocompatibility complex (MHC) class II and helps the immune system distinguish self-proteins from foreign invaders. But having even two copies of the 'bad' gene only confers an 8.3-fold increased risk,[13] so there is no single 'MS gene' and there is no genetic test for MS.

Luckily, although our genes are a risk factor for getting MS, there is no strong genetic effect on the course of MS. The risk genes in people with benign and aggressive MS are similar, and people with primary progressive MS have no greater 'genetic load' (number of risk genes) than those with relapsing MS.[14] It is common for two close relatives to have dramatically different disease courses, even for identical twins![15] Indeed, there is powerful evidence that

Table 1.2: Approximate risk of MS in relatives

Type of relative	Risk of developing MS
Identical (monozygotic) twin (100% genetic relatedness)	17–25%
Fraternal (dizygotic) twin (50% genetic relatedness)	2–5%
Parent, sibling, child (1° relative, 50% genetic relatedness)	1–3%
Aunt/uncle/niece/nephew/half-sibling (2° relatives, 25% genetic relatedness)	1%
Cousins (3° relative, 12.5% relatedness)	0.4%
Adopted child (unrelated)	0.4%
Unrelated (background risk in the United States)	0.3%

Note: As I used multiple sources, I rounded to the nearest whole number or gave a range. Comparison between the different percentages is limited as not all sources analysed all types of relatives. As yet we do not know the extent to which lifestyle changes modify these statistics.

MS is largely driven by environmental risk factors. After all, the prevalence of MS varies dramatically by region. It is one in 222 in Syracuse, New York (USA),[16] but only one in 25,000 in Cuenca, Ecuador![17] Ecuadorians are genetically similar to Hispanics in the United States, who have a similar risk to Europeans.[18, 19]

Some environmental factors are difficult to control. For example, being born in the spring months is a slight risk factor for MS, possibly because of lower levels of vitamin D during the mother's pregnancy that occurred mostly throughout winter. MS is also linked to Epstein Barr Virus (EBV), a virus that causes 'mononucleosis' (glandular fever) but often causes no symptoms. EBV is everywhere and has infected over 90 per cent of people worldwide,[20] usually during childhood or adolescence. Nearly all people with MS have evidence of prior EBV exposure,[21] and avoiding it may be impossible.

The prevalence of MS across different countries and even within countries varies greatly

We also see more MS in developed countries, and some research- ers believe modern hygiene, and in particular the absence of parasite infections during youth, may derange the immune system and pre- dispose people to autoimmune disease.[22] Needless to say, genes and certain environmental risk factors are out of our control.

However, we also know that modifiable environmental risk factors are important. We see the prevalence of MS rising every- where in the world. Regions where MS was historically rare, such as India, Iran and Mexico, are now seeing frequent cases. I have spoken with older international neurologists at professional con- ferences who assure me this is not simply increasing recognition. MS is challenging to diagnose, but it strikes early enough and is dramatic enough to be very apparent to local doctors in these countries. The only plausible explanation is that modern lifestyles associated with 'Westernisation' are causing the disease.

It seems that a 'perfect storm' of environmental factors must occur in a genetically susceptible host for MS to develop and progress. The genetically susceptible person may develop MS when exposed to certain environmental factors. Some of these factors, as discussed, are unavoidable, but I will introduce a few lifestyle behaviour modifications that can reduce a susceptible individual's risk of developing the illness. We will learn further details about these modifiable risk factors in future chapters. The simplest example is smoking, which increases the risk of MS and speeds its progression. To a smoker with MS, quitting is the first and simplest advice I give.

Sunlight and vitamin D

Sunlight exposure is a significant consideration in addition to smoking. The risk of MS increases with distance from the equator as ultraviolet light exposure gets naturally lower (Figure 1.5). And within individual countries such as Australia, England, Sweden and the United States, the risk also varies with latitude; in Australia, for example, MS is six times more common in southern Tasmania (furthest from the equator) than Queensland in the north (closer to the equator). When there are two identical twins, and one has MS

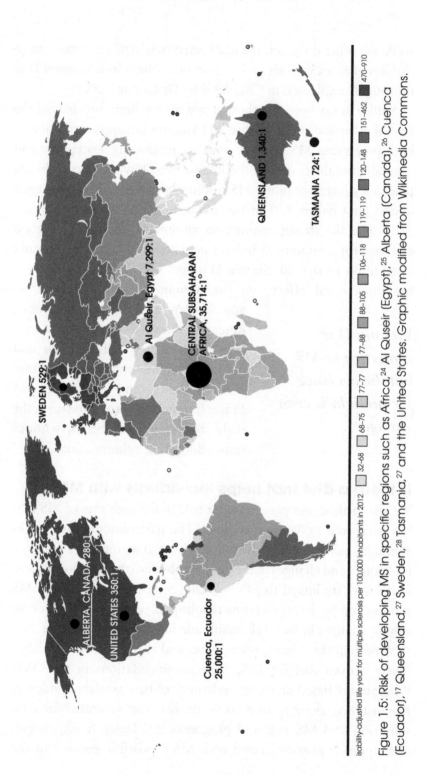

Figure 1.5: Risk of developing MS in specific regions such as Africa,[24] Al Quseir (Egypt),[24] Alberta (Canada),[25] Cuenca (Ecuador),[17] Queensland,[27] Sweden,[28] Tasmania,[27] and the United States. Graphic modified from Wikimedia Commons.

QUEENSLAND 1,340:1

TASMANIA 724:1

Al Quseir, Egypt 7,299:1

CENTRAL SUBSAHARAN AFRICA, 35,714:1

SWEDEN 529:1

ALBERTA, CANADA 280:1

UNITED STATES 350:1

Cuenca, Ecuador 25,000:1

Disability-adjusted life year for multiple sclerosis per 100,000 inhabitants in 2012 32–68 68–75 77–77 77–88 88–105 106–118 119–119 120–148 151–462 470–910 while the other does not, the unaffected twin tends to report more childhood sun exposure.[23] The role of sunlight and vitamin D is thoroughly explained in Chapter 4 by Dr Conor Kerley.

Suffice to say here that there is now strong literature around the role of adequate sun exposure and vitamin D supplementation in both preventing MS in those who are genetically susceptible and in modifying the course of the illness. Even low vitamin D during pregnancy increases future MS risk for the child.[29] This is discussed in detail in Chapter 9, 'Families and prevention'.

Despite the strong research on vitamin D, there is very good evidence for a vitamin-D-independent effect of sunlight exposure in addition to that of vitamin D alone. UV light exposure itself has unexpected effects on the immune system, a phenomenon known as 'photoimmunology'. Research shows that sunlight stimulates suppressor T-cell function and induces anti-inflammatory cytokines such as IL-10 and IL-4.[30] It also causes immune tolerance, meaning the body 'tolerates' itself better, without responding with inflammation.

Vitamin D is protective in MS, but the evidence for sunlight is even stronger

Is there a diet that helps individuals with MS?

We also believe diet plays a major role in the high rate of MS that has been seen in Western nations. The gastrointestinal tract has abundant gut-associated lymphoid tissue that regulates immune function,[31] and changes in the gut microbiome (the microorganisms in the gut) are linked to MS.[32, 33] One compelling theory says MS is provoked by deranged fat metabolism as people with the disease exhibit changes in their cell membrane fatty acid composition.[34]

Although the science is complex, and there is no single definitively proven diet for MS, the recommendations in the OMS Program are based on a preponderance of best available evidence. For instance, there is an association between saturated fat consumption and MS risk and prognosis.[35-37] Dairy (milk, cheese, and so on) is also connected with MS,[38] possibly because of the milk protein butyrophilin, which may trigger an immune response against myelin.[39] High intake of salt, abundant in processed foods, may be another factor.[40] The next Part, 'The directions', provides detailed and explicit lifestyle advice for MS.

Saturated fat, dairy and salt intake correlates with MS risk

What is the standard medical treatment for MS?

For acute MS attacks, steroids can help speed recovery. Common regimens in adults are 1000 milligrams intravenous Solumedrol© (methylprednisolone) or 1250 milligrams oral prednisone daily for 3–5 days. For severe relapses that do not improve with steroids, a dialysis-like procedure called plasma exchange can remove antibodies and inflammatory cytokines, sometimes leading to improvement.

In the long run, medications referred to as 'disease-modifying therapies' (DMTs) can help prevent attacks and new MRI lesions. They are for relapse prevention and do not necessarily improve the symptoms of MS, just like aspirin may lower risk of a second heart attack but does not reduce damage from the first heart attack. The DMTs approved by the US and European regulatory authorities in 2020 are summarised in Table 1.3, and other MS drugs are shown in Table 1.4. All of these drugs reduce the rate of attacks and development of new MRI lesions, and for some of the drugs there is additional evidence for reduction in long-term disability and brain atrophy.

A detailed discussion of the mechanisms, clinical trials data, and risk-benefit analysis of these medications is constantly evolving and beyond the scope of this book. This is a topic best left to your own research and a trusted medical adviser, although Chapter 7 on medications by Dr Jonathan White goes into a bit more detail than is possible here. There is evidence that early initiation of high-efficacy DMTs for young people with relapsing MS yields the greatest success. However, the more effective therapies have greater risks, and none has been trialled in conjunction with lifestyle modification.

Table 1.3: FDA/EMA-approved DMTs for MS, showing the trade and generic names, route of administration, and common side effects

Drug (brand name)	Generic name	Route	Common side effects
Betaseron© Extavia©	beta-interferon 1b	Subcutaneous injection every other day	Muscle aches, flu-like symptoms, liver injury
Rebif©	beta-interferon 1a	Subcutaneous injection three times weekly	Muscle aches, flu-like symptoms, liver injury
Avonex©	beta-interferon 1a	Intramuscular injection once weekly	Muscle aches, flu-like symptoms, liver injury
Plegridy©	beta-interferon 1a	Intramuscular injection once per 2 weeks	Muscle aches, flu-like symptoms, liver injury
Copaxone© Glatopa©	glatiramer acetate	Subcutaneous injection daily or three times a week	Injection site reactions, skin dimpling
Gilenya©	fingolimod	Orally daily	Slow heart rate, infections, macular edema
Mayzent©	siponimod	Orally daily	Slow heart rate, infections, macular edema
Zeposia©	ozanimod	Orally daily	Slow heart rate, infections, macular edema
Tecfidera©	dimethyl fumarate	Orally twice daily	Skin flushing, infections, diarrhoea
Vumerity©	diroximel fumarate	Orally twice daily	Skin flushing, infections, diarrhoea

Bafiertam©	Monomethyl fumarate	Orally twice daily	Skin flushing, infections, diarrhoea
Aubagio©	teriflunomide	Orally daily	Diarrhoea, hair loss, infections
Tysabri©	natalizumab	Monthly infusion	Allergic reaction, progressive multifocal leukoencephalopathy (rare brain infection)
Ocrevus©	ocrelizumab	Infusion every six months	Allergic reaction, infections
Kesimpta©	ofatumumab	Subcutaneous injection monthly	Allergic reaction, infections
Lemtrada©	alemtuzumab	Infusion (variable number of cycles)	Allergic reaction, infections, secondary autoimmune diseases
Novantrone©	mitoxantrone	Infusion every 3 months	Infections, heart failure, leukaemia
Mavenclad©	cladribine	Orally with variable dosing	Nausea, hair loss, infections

Table 1.4: 'Off-label' (not formally approved for MS by regulatory agencies) DMTs, showing the trade and generic names, route of administration, and common side effects

Drug (brand name)	Generic name	Route	Common side effects
Rituxan©	rituximab	Infusion every 6 months	Allergic reaction, infections
Arzerra©	ofatumumab	Infusion every 6 months	Allergic reaction, infections
Arava©	leflunomide	Orally daily	Diarrhoea, hair loss, infections
Imuran©	azathioprine	Orally twice daily	Gastrointestinal upset, infections
Cytoxan©	cyclophosphamide	Monthly infusion or orally	Hair loss, infections, bladder injury, infertility
Rheumatrex©	methotrexate	Orally weekly	Gastrointestinal upset, infections
Leustatin©	cladribine	Intravenous (undefined dosing)	Nausea, hair loss, infections
Cellcept©	mycophenolate mofetil	Orally twice daily	Gastrointestinal upset, infections
Zocor©	simvastatin	Orally daily	Muscle aches, liver injury
N/A	biotin (vitamin B7)	300mg orally daily	Abnormal lab test results (TSH, troponin)
Minocin©	minocycline	Orally twice daily	Gastrointestinal upset, rash, dental discolouration, dizziness
N/A	ibudilast	Orally daily	Gastrointestinal upset, headache, depression
N/A	Haematopoietic Stem Cell Transplant (HSCT). Various agents (e.g. cyclophosphamide, anti-thymocyte globulin, busulfan, BEAM)	Variable	Immunosuppression, anaemia, bladder toxicity, infertility, other

Note: An HSCT to treat MS can use various 'conditioning' regimens, each with unique effectiveness and risk.

There are many drugs for MS called 'disease-modifying therapies' (DMTs) that can help prevent relapses and new MRI lesions; some have been shown to reduce brain shrinkage and disability progression

Besides management of acute attacks and long-term prevention with DMTs, there are 'symptomatic' treatments for MS. These are medications or other interventions that treat a variety of chronic symptoms, such as bladder problems, fatigue, pain, depression, tremor or gait difficulty. An example is treating muscle spasticity with massage, physical therapy and the drug baclofen. Every person is unique and will face different challenges, so we often need a personalised approach rather than a one-size-fits-all solution.

Regardless of your specific challenges, now is a better time than it ever has been to be diagnosed with MS. We have more treatments, technology and information than ever before, and a worldwide MS community that shares its experience and guidance. When you are ill, confused and scared, it is easy to accept treatment passively. But you must remember, you are your own best advocate. Only you can fully understand the symptoms you experience. Only you can decide whether to accept the risk of a particular treatment. Only you can commit to making the lifestyle changes that will maximise your long-term health. Do not underestimate the power you have over your life.

The MS road may have many curves and potholes, challenging you to make difficult decisions and, at times, sacrifices, but it may also encourage you to exercise new abilities or find new opportunities. Some with MS discover within themselves talents and resilience that previously lay dormant. Onyeka was stunned when she first received her diagnosis, but I am happy to report she is doing well both physically and emotionally, and she is more determined and adventurous than ever before. I hope this book gives you the confidence, energy and enthusiasm needed to make lifelong changes so you can live the life you were meant to live.

Ground covered

MS is sometimes called the 'snowflake disease' because it affects each person uniquely. Some report no symptoms while others are plagued by disabilities both conspicuous and invisible. In truth, many people do much better for much longer than the general population expects, yet subtle changes over time can be life-changing, career-derailing and relationship-straining.

Although we think of it as a mysterious, unexplained and unpredictable disease (which it is), it is empowering to know that lifestyle plays a very important role in its genesis and course. Like much of life, the quality of our health can sometimes come down to luck, but the evidence for an environmental component in the development and course of MS is unquestionable. The low prevalence of MS near the equator and in developing countries shows us that modern society, sunlight and culture are all factors impacting on the disease. The epidemiologic evidence for the role of vitamin D, saturated fat and dairy is also quite strong.

We can learn from patients like Onyeka, ignoring what is beyond our control and focusing on what we can change. A wise person will utilise everything available: the marvels of modern medicine, support and information from a global community, and simple everyday choices.

References

1. 'MS on the rise in Australia but still flying under our radar', *MS Research Australia*, 1 May 2018, <https://msra.org.au/news/ms-rise-australia-still-flying-radar/>, accessed 19 April 2021.

2. Culpepper, W.J., Marrie, R.A., Langer-Gould, A. et al., 'Validation of an algorithm for identifying MS cases in administrative health claims data-bases', *Neurology*, 2019, 92(10).

3. Andravizou, A., Dardiotis, E., Artemiadis, A. et al., 'Brain atrophy in multiple sclerosis: Mechanisms, clinical relevance and treatment options', *Autoimmune Highlights*, 2019, 10(7).

4. Kappos, L, Wolinsky, J.S., Giovannoni, G. et al., 'Contribution of relapse-independent progression vs relapse-associated worsening to overall confirmed disability accumulation in typical relapsing multiple sclerosis in

a pooled analysis of 2 randomized clinical trials', *JAMA Neurology*, 2020, 77(9): 1–9.

5. Siva, A., 'Asymptomatic MS', *Clinical Neurology and Neurosurgery*, 2013, 115, Suppl 1: S1–S5.

6. University of California, San Francisco MS-EPIC Team: Cree, B.A.C., Gourraud, P.A., Oksenberg, J.R. et al., 'Long-term evolution of multiple sclerosis disability in the treatment era', *Annals of Neurology*, 2016, 80(4): 499–510.

7. Miller, D.H., Hornabrook, R.W. & Purdie, G., 'The natural history of multiple sclerosis: A regional study with some longitudinal data', *Journal of Neurology, Neurosurgery and Psychiatry*, 1992, 55: 341–46.

8. Beiki, O., Frumento, P., Bottai, M., Manouchehrinia, A. & Hillert, J., 'Changes in the risk of reaching multiple sclerosis disability milestones in recent decades: A nationwide population-based cohort study in Sweden', *JAMA Neurology*, 2019; 76(6): 665–71.

9. Jongen, P.J., Ter Horst, A.T. & Brands, A.M., 'Cognitive impairment in multiple sclerosis', *Minerva Medica*, 2012, 103(2): 73–96.

10. Willis, S.N. & Stathopoulos, P., 'Investigating the antigen specificity of multiple sclerosis central nervous system-derived immunoglobulins', *Frontiers in Immunology*, 2015, 6: 600.

11. Frischer, J.M., Weigand, S.D., Guo, Y. et al., 'Clinical and pathological insights into the dynamic nature of the white matter multiple sclerosis plaque', *Annals of Neurology*, 2015, 78(5): 710–21.

12. Absinta, M., Lassmann, H. & Trapp, B.D., 'Mechanisms underlying progression in multiple sclerosis', *Current Opinion in Neurology*, 2020, 33(3): 277–85.

13. Alcina, A., Abad-Grau, M. & Fedetz, M., 'Multiple sclerosis risk variant HLA-DRB1*1501 associates with high expression of DRB1 gene in different human populations', *PLoS One*, 2012, 7(1): e29819.

14. McDonnell, G.V., Mawhinney, H., Graham, C.A., Hawkins, S.A. & Middleton, D. 'A study of the HLA-DR region in clinical subgroups of multiple sclerosis and its influence on prognosis', *Journal of the Neurological Sciences*, 1999, 165(1): 77–83.

15. Williams, A., Eldridge, R., McFarland, H., Houff, S., Krebs, H. & McFarlin, D., 'Multiple sclerosis in twins', *Neurology*, 1980, 30(11): 1139–47.

16. Sladek, T., 'The MS mystery in Syracuse: Why do we have highest rate of multiple sclerosis nationwide?', 5 November 2019, *CNY Central*, <https://cnycentral.com/news/local/the-ms-mystery-in-syracuse-why-do-we-have-highest-rate-of-multiple-sclerosis-nationwide>, accessed July 2020.

17. Correa-Díaz, E.P. & Ortiz, M.A., 'Prevalence of multiple sclerosis in Cuenca, Ecuador', *Multiple Sclerosis Journal—Experimental, transnational and clinical*, 2019, 5(4).

18. Zambrano, A.K. & Gaviria, A., 'The three-hybrid genetic composition of an Ecuadorian population using AIMs-InDels compared with autosomes, mitochondrial DNA and Y chromosome data', *Scientific Reports*, 2019, 9, 9247.

19. Langer-Gould, A., Brara, S.M., Beaber, B.E. & Zhang, J.L., 'Incidence of multiple sclerosis in multiple racial and ethnic groups', *Neurology*, 2013, 80(19): 1734–39.

20. Smatti, M.K., Al-Sadeq, D.W. & Ali, N.H. et al., 'Epstein-Barr Virus epidemiology, serology, and genetic variability of LMP-1 oncogene among healthy population: An update', *Frontiers in Oncology*, 13 June 2018.

21. Guan, Y., Jakimovski, D., Ramanathan, M. et al., 'The role of Epstein-Barr virus in multiple sclerosis: From molecular pathophysiology to in vivo imaging', *Neural Regeneration Research*, 2019, 14(3): 373–86.

22. Ascherio, A. et al., 'The initiation and prevention of multiple sclerosis', *Nature Reviews Neurology*, 2012, 8(11): 602–12.

23. Islam, T., Gauderman, J.W., Cozen, W. & Mack, T.M., 'Childhood sun exposure influences risk of multiple sclerosis in monozygotic twins', *Neurology*, 2007, 69(4): 381–88.

24. GBD 2016 Multiple Sclerosis Collaborators, 'Global, regional, and national burden of multiple sclerosis 1990–2016: Systematic analysis for the global burden of disease study 2016', *The Lancet, Neurology*, 2019, 18(3): 269–85.

25. El-Tallawy, H.N. et al., 'Prevalence of multiple sclerosis in Al Quseir city, Red Sea Governorate, Egypt', *Neuropsychiatric Disease and Treatment*, 2016, 12: 155–8.

26. Amankwah, N. et al., 'Multiple sclerosis in Canada 2011 to 2031: Results of a microsimulation modelling study of epidemiological and economic impacts'. 'La sclérose en plaques au Canada, 2011–2031: Résultats d'une étude de modélisation par microsimulation des répercussions épidémiologiques et économiques', *Health Promotion and Chronic Disease Prevention in Canada: Research, policy and practice*, 2017, 37(2): 37–48.

27. Campbell, J.A., Simpson, S. Jr, Ahmad, H., Taylor, B.V., van der Mei, I. & Palmer, A.J., 'Change in multiple sclerosis prevalence over time in Australia 2010–2017 utilising disease-modifying therapy prescription data', *Multiple Sclerosis*, 2020, 26(11): 1315–28.

28. Ahlgren, C., Odén, A. & Lycke, J., 'High nationwide prevalence of multiple sclerosis in Sweden', *Multiple Sclerosis*, 2011, 17(8): 901–8.

29. Mirzaei, F. et al., 'Gestational vitamin D and the risk of multiple sclerosis in offspring', *Annals of Neurology*, 2011, 70(1): 30–40.

30. Paz, L.M. et al., 'Time-course evaluation and treatment of skin inflammatory immune response after ultraviolet B irradiation', *Cytokine*, 2008, 44(1): 70–7.

31. Brandtzaeg P., Valnes, K., Scott, H., Rognum, T.O., Bjerke, K. & Baklien, K., 'The human gastrointestinal secretory immune system in health and disease', *Scandinavian Journal of Gastroenterology Supplement*, 1985: 114: 17–38.

32. Jhangi, S., Gandhi, R. et al., 'Increased archaea species and changes with therapy in gut microbiome of multiple sclerosis subjects', *Neurology*, 2014, 82(10 Supplement): S24.00.

33. Farrokhi, V. et al., 'Bacterial lipodipeptide, Lipid 654, is a microbiome-associated biomarker for multiple sclerosis', *Clinical and Translational Immunology*, 2013, 2(11): e8. 15.

34. Baker, R.W., Thompson, R.H. & Zilkha, K.J., 'Fatty-acid composition of brain lecithins in multiple sclerosis', *Lancet*, 1963, 1(7271): 26–7.

35. Azary S., Schreiner T., Graves J. et al., 'Contribution of dietary intake to relapse rate in early paediatric multiple sclerosis', *Journal of Neurology, Neurosurgery and Psychiatry*, 2018, 89: 28–33.

36. Swank, R.L., Lerstad, O., Strøm, A. & Backer, J., 'Multiple sclerosis in rural Norway: Its geographic and occupational incidence in relation to nutrition', *New England Journal of Medicine*, 1952, 246(19): 722–8.

37. Swank, R.L., 'Multiple sclerosis: A correlation of its incidence with dietary fat', *American Journal of Medical Science*, 1950, 220(4): 421–30.

38. Munger, K.L., Chitnis, T., Frazier, A.L., Giovannucci, E., Spiegelman, D. & Ascherio, A., 'Dietary intake of vitamin D during adolescence and risk of multiple sclerosis', *Journal of Neurology*, 2011, 258(3): 479–85.

39. Stefferl, A., Schubart, A., Storch M. et al., 'Butyrophilin, a milk protein, modulates the encephalitogenic T cell response to myelin oligodendrocyte glycoprotein in experimental autoimmune encephalomyelitis', *Journal of Immunology*, 2000, 165(5): 2859–65.

40. Farez, M.F., Fiol, M.P., Gaitán, M.I., Quintana, F.J. & Correale, J., 'Sodium intake is associated with increased disease activity in multiple sclerosis', *Journal of Neurology, Neurosurgery and Psychiatry*, 2015, 86(1): 26–31.

Part 2

The directions

2

Overview of the OMS Program

Dr Virginia Billson

It feels like I have found a new friend in the OMS Program, allowing me to take control and lead a more healthy and positive life. Bravo!

Clare McKenzie, Burnham-on-Crouch, UK, OMSer

My diagnosis of MS was a mixed blessing in 1996, confirmed as it was by an MRI scan and spinal fluid, blood and visual field tests on my 47th birthday. At least my visual and physical symptoms were not those of a malignant brain tumour, a stroke or any of the other ghastly conditions that I, as a medical specialist pathologist, was aware of and feared. At the same time, so many unexpected and potentially life-changing questions leaped into my rather shocked and addled brain. Were there any successful treatments for MS? Would I be disabled soon? Would I have to cease my dearly loved career? What would become of my active family and social lives?

I developed a bleak outlook after spending two intense months reading a mountain of medical texts and journals. I decided then to pretty much give up researching the topic. I was feeling quite well after a heavy course of prednisone, which, apart from a few slight sensory symptoms, resolved my double vision and leg weakness. I resolved to forget about MS, ignore the reality of my diagnosis and get on with my busy life. However, the reality of MS wouldn't be suppressed or ignored. What followed were four years of a wild roller-coaster of attacks, which included weird symptoms, and increasing fatigue and depression, all of which viciously interrupted many aspects of my previously rewarding and rich family, social and professional lives.

And then, at a People with MS Christmas party, I was recommended a book to read that was written by an Australian doctor with MS. It was the very first edition of *Taking Control of Multiple Sclerosis* by Professor George Jelinek. It was a revelation. The book described things I could do for myself to regain control over the disease and improve all aspects of my health and life, which I had felt I was losing a grip on every day. The book outlined a lifestyle program that was based on very convincing scientific evidence and principles that I could buy into, no airy-fairy, hippy-trippy ideas but hard data. And so started my twenty-year adventure slowly incorporating the methods and principles of *Taking Control of Multiple Sclerosis*, which eventually developed into the OMS Program.

What is the OMS Program and where does it fit into our day-to-day lives?

The 21st century is a time of wondrous advances in our daily lives. We can travel to the other side of the world in a day or two (pandemics permitting), we can get into our cars and travel for hundreds of kilometres in a few hours, we can use technology to interact with friends and colleagues around the globe in a matter of minutes, we live longer than our forebears, and medical treatments can cure or alleviate many infectious and other diseases.

It has long been said, initially by Sir Isaac Newton in his laws of motion in 1686, that 'for every action there is an equal and opposite reaction' and along with our incredible advances we unfortunately have had to deal with many negative environmental, social, physical and mental effects.

In the developed world, the fast-paced lives we lead make getting enough exercise and quiet contemplation quite a challenge.

The busy days seduce us with easily obtained and highly processed fast foods and make us seek 'instant' gratification through sweets and salty snacks. Eating out frequently at cafes and restaurants enables us to overeat too many rich meals to 'get our money's worth'. Excessive alcohol intake, overuse of prescription and illegal drugs and cigarette smoking are also easily indulged in. Increased stress as a result of our high-pressure jobs and rapidly changing environment adds to the burden of illness.

We often neglect our wellbeing and consume too much of the wrong foods, are lax about exercising and disregard the value of quiet pondering or just thinking and appreciating what we have, not what we could purchase if we earned more money.

As a consequence of these habits that we have so readily incorporated into our daily lives, there has been an epidemic of lifestyle-related health problems, such as type 2 diabetes, cardiovascular disease, some common cancers, respiratory impairment and obesity, to name just a few. We know that these ailments are major risk factors for a host of further disorders, such as sleep disturbances including sleep apnoea, muscle and joint problems and, as shown by recent research, a higher incidence of Alzheimer's disease and other dementias.

It is getting harder and harder to stay well in the 21st century, despite, or sometimes because of, all the advances we have made

Each of the lifestyle diseases mentioned can spiral into further complications requiring medical or even surgical intervention and their often-intrusive side effects. MS, which is increasing in incidence, has been identified as being one such disorder on the long and growing list of lifestyle-related diseases.

The OMS Program is based on sound scientific principles and research and is able to be accessed by anyone with MS. This combination of lifestyle adjustments, when embraced as a whole, has been shown to complement or, in some people, replace the need for medications, and to vastly improve the condition or even reverse some of the symptoms. Adopting and persisting with the recommended lifestyle changes as part of a healthy approach to the rest of your life certainly requires active engagement with the philosophy and details of OMS. Incorporating the OMS recommendations into a daily routine requires some research, understanding, trust and belief, and only when it becomes part of daily life can you slowly but surely feel the benefits to MS and general health.

The OMS Program is based on sound scientific principles and research

I will give a very brief overview of what the OMS Program is about—more detail on each aspect and other relevant issues will be expanded in the following chapters.

Let's start with diet

Research has consistently shown that the modern Western diet contains large quantities of saturated fats, which come mainly from animal sources, and relatively low quantities of fibre and nutrients, especially the B group vitamins and omega-3 fatty acids. This type of diet promotes the hardening of arteries, with the consequence of an increasing incidence of heart disease and stroke. Saturated fats stimulate inflammation throughout the body and increase the chances of getting various types of cancer, among a host of other diseases.

As described by Dr Beaber in Chapter 1, MS is largely a disorder of an overactive immune system, also known as an autoimmune disorder, which leads to inflammation in the brain and spinal cord that in turn causes the many and varied symptoms with which we are all familiar: loss or blurring of vision, weakness in parts of the muscular system such as your legs, sensations of numbness or tingling, and nerve pain are fairly common. These can to a large extent be improved by the OMS Program, which includes a change in diet that eliminates as much saturated fat as possible. Eating a mainly plant-based and high-fibre range of fresh foods is both nourishing and, using the many cooking resources now available, can be delicious. Supplementing the diet with foods rich in omega-3 fatty acids, as found in fish, seafood and flaxseeds and their oils, has been also associated with better outcomes for people with MS. Supplementation with B group vitamins may also be beneficial in some circumstances.

A major change of diet involving restriction or elimination of many of the foods we previously considered normal can be quite daunting and sadly can turn many people off the Program. Some people find that modifying aspects of their dietary regime fairly gradually, and approaching the whole task with curiosity and interest, can make the changes a satisfying objective, especially since they have been proven to have huge benefits. Other people find they are more successful when they actively and rapidly embrace all aspects of modifying their diet.

How we manage the changes depends on each individual's personality and their approach to major life hurdles. It can, however, be a real adventure to experiment with new ways of preparing our food and research new recipes to produce delicious, satisfying and wholesome meals.

Changing to an ultra-healthy diet can be a really enjoyable adventure

Encouraging your nearest and dearest to join in the food adventure can have fantastic health benefits for you and everyone in the family, as the dietary recommendations have been shown to reduce many of our Western ailments and potentially reduce the possibility of your genetically related family members from developing MS (see Jack McNulty's views on diet in Chapter 3 and read more detail about family issues in Chapter 9).

Another important aspect of the OMS diet is the avoidance of dairy products. There are two major reasons to avoid the breast milk of other animals such as cows: the fat is largely saturated and therefore unhealthy, and proteins in milk may also cause problems for people with MS or with a predisposition to developing MS. The structure of cow's milk protein is very similar to human myelin, the fatty insulating coating of our nerves, which is the target of the inflammatory attack in MS. Consuming dairy products may cause the body to react to this milk protein—the effect can then spill over and become part of the damaging autoimmune reaction to our own myelin. Elimination of dairy products is strongly recommended and we are fortunate today that there are many plant-based alternatives that are as nutritionally wholesome as cow's milk and quite delicious too.

On a more positive note, alcohol in moderation does not seem to be harmful for people with MS and a glass of wine with our thoughtfully cooked meal can be enjoyed as a real reward for a job well done.

Sunshine and its vitamin—vitamin D

Epidemiological studies over many decades and in numerous countries have pointed to the fact that low sun exposure can predispose the population to an increase in the incidence of MS. In Chapter 4, Dr Conor Kerley outlines how the sun reacts with chemicals in the skin to produce vitamin D3. This vitamin has many vital roles in the body, including the maintenance of strong bones and muscles and preventing the disabling bone disease called rickets. How vitamin D reacts with the immune system is of crucial importance to those of us with MS. Appropriate vitamin D blood levels can moderate or balance the immune system so that it reduces a hyperactive immune system without suppressing it.

Both sunshine and the vitamin D it produces in the body are helpful for people with MS and their families, but be mindful of getting too much sun exposure

Sun exposure, and in particular the UVB rays of the sun, has also been shown to act as an immune modulator independent of the vitamin D effects, so direct sunlight is thought to be useful in combination with vitamin D. Of course, we have to be mindful of the harmful effects of too much sun in any sunny environment. Skin cancer is a lethal consequence that we all want to strenuously avoid. How to get just the right and safe amount is described in detail in Chapter 4.

Get enough of the right sort of exercise

In past decades, exercise was not considered an important part of the management of MS. In many cases it was actively discouraged and people with MS became increasingly weak and disabled. There is now abundant evidence that regular aerobic exercise to build cardiovascular fitness and strength-building exercises are of utmost importance for people living with many chronic diseases, including MS.

Research into the effects of exercise on diabetes, cardiovascular disease, high blood pressure and many cancers has shown clear-cut benefits. The research has also shown that regular exercise in people who are living with these conditions results in improvements in many aspects of their quality of life, in particular their mental health. They are happier, have better cognitive abilities such as memory, and often have much improved outcomes for their underlying disease.

Exercise is important in a number of ways. The prospect of losing mobility is one of the most painful fears that people with MS live with every day. Exercise together with the other components of the OMS Program can slow or even reverse a person's physical limitations. Exercise is well known to make people feel better and 'runner's high' is a recognised characteristic that many vigorous exercisers experience. Moderate exercise can also make you feel more optimistic and joyful, which can improve your mental outlook. In many people exercise can lift a person's mood and decrease the frequency and severity of depression. Dr Stuart White goes into this in a lot more detail in Chapter 5.

Physical exercise can also decrease the incidence of a number of the other Western scourges obesity, diabetes, osteoporosis and cancer.

Exercise is beneficial for people with MS in a host of different ways; it is an essential part of the OMS Program

Fatigue is a very common, disabling and often invisible symptom in people with MS. It can reduce one's enjoyment of daily life and is known to be an influencing factor for many of us deciding to limit or stop paid or voluntary work and curtail social and family activities. Exercise in MS has been shown to alleviate fatigue and increase endurance and this 'side effect' can be extremely powerful.

Exercise can also improve our balance, strength and stability, and in turn reduce the incidence of falls. Even small falls can lead to significant injuries that can severely impact on the ability to manage at home or at work. Exercises building muscular strength can also decrease the development of osteoporosis or 'brittle bones'. Together with general bodily weakness and impaired balance, osteoporosis can lead to bone fragility and fractures. Loss of function and movement is to be strenuously avoided if possible.

And remember the mind–body connection

The mind is a powerful thing. For millennia the impact of the mind on bodily functions and ailments has been increasingly recognised. The mind is known to be responsible for both positive and negative aspects of health, physical as well as mental. External influences like the loss of loved ones or even worldwide disasters, such as pandemics, can lead to severe stress reactions. Even the anticipation of having to sit for an exam, give a speech, perform in front of a crowd or attend an interview can be so stressful as to reduce some of us to the point of tears and even total shutdown. Research has shown that for those living with MS, stress can have profound effects and can trigger an MS attack or relapse.

Many physicians recommend their patients 'de-stress' their lives to assist them in recovering from a range of physical and mental disorders. Unfortunately, advice on how to develop the tools to undertake this often complex task is often lacking. Although psychologists and counsellors skilled in assisting people with chronic diseases can be a valuable aid in helping someone to de-stress, being in control of your own mental strength and having the ability to manage your stress levels with the regular practice of meditation or other mindfulness-based strategies can be empowering and can build self-recovery. Internationally renowned mindfulness expert Associate Professor Craig Hassed goes into this in detail in Chapter 6. Don't underestimate the power of the simple techniques he outlines.

I have had many discussions with people with MS over the years in my role as a peer support worker and MS Ambassador, and meditation appears to be one of the OMS strategies that many of us find the most difficult to incorporate into daily life. It is not a natural action to withdraw from often busy lives and actively focus attention elsewhere for a period of time. There are, however, many techniques and online resources available to help people learn to meditate and that can be gradually introduced into day-to-day life. Once I absorbed the large evidence base that describes the profound positive effects that regular meditation can provide, it was much easier to accept some techniques that I could practise regularly and even to enjoy regular meditation. This is a form of therapy with only positive side effects and is one we can implement without a prescription or a pill.

And finally, what part does medication play?

The OMS Program is one that can and does work well together with any prescribed medications from your doctor. Some of the new raft of medicines that have become available to treat mainly the relapsing and remitting forms of MS unfortunately can have many disturbing side effects. Many people with MS have been able to successfully reduce their dependence on medications, under the supervision of their supportive medical practitioner, away from requiring medication to stay well just by strictly adhering to the OMS lifestyle recommendations. Others such as myself choose the 'belt and braces' approach: I have continued with my relatively low-impact medication for over twenty years while following the OMS Program. Still others looking to do whatever it takes to minimise the effects of MS in their lives opt for one of the more recently released potent medications. The OMS approach works very well as a complement to other treatments and does not interfere with or complicate them. Dr Jonathan White goes into the issues involved in choosing a disease-modifying therapy in Chapter 7.

Other considerations

Starting a new way of approaching a chronic condition that is going to impact health and daily life can be an initially unsettling prospect, especially for those recently diagnosed and trying to navigate a storm of scary emotions. This book and a couple of other OMS-themed books can set you on a positive road to healing and recovery. Even more powerful is a group retreat or workshop that promotes the lifestyle recommendations discussed above. This may be especially useful early in your travels along this sometimes bumpy highway. The group settings are unfortunately not widely available around the world but researching your own locale to see if one is in reach is strongly encouraged. Two retreats I attended a few years apart were a revelation for me and made the recommendations in the book so much more approachable and understandable. Meeting together with other people with MS who were dealing with the wide range of issues that I was dealing with myself was both reassuring and comforting, and having direct access to the professionals running the course was incredible. Being able to question any and every aspect of the OMS Program was motivating and engaging, so I urge you to do it if you can.

Stop smoking if you are a smoker and avoid a second-hand smoke environment if your household has smokers in it. Extensive research has shown that the contents of tobacco smoke are especially toxic to people with MS and can predispose individuals to initially developing MS and its subsequent progression. There are no positive side effects of smoking and it should be strongly discouraged, especially in the household and around genetically related family members.

There are many resources available to help people with MS adopt the OMS Program

Dealing with all aspects of health and management of MS requires a team of both professionals and personal contacts to whom you can easily relate. The team needs to include people who can understand your needs and assist you in being your best self. Some doctors have been quite dismissive of the benefits of the OMS approach. They may not have carefully researched the mountains of evidence that are accumulating on the benefits of the individual components of the Program.

Combining all the aspects of the OMS Program discussed earlier is both powerful and achievable and within your control. So select your team well (Dr Heather King talks about this in detail in Chapter 11) and you may have to educate them too, as I had to. Even some senior professors either hadn't heard of the Program or were quite negative about its potential benefits. I distributed the first book quite widely among my medical colleagues and I think I converted many of them, especially when they took the trouble to absorb all the current scientific data that is accumulating.

It is probably even more important to have a small, easily accessed support group on your team that may be family, friends or people with MS who are peers and who also follow the OMS Program. These people need to be aware of how you are going, able to support you emotionally, and willing to join you on this long adventurous road to being your best self. The internet can be a valuable part of your support but be aware of the various traps and destructive aspects of this source of information. I have accessed a number of sites but have found some to be quite distressing and even dangerous, with dubious (and often expensive) advice sometimes being promoted. Starting with the OMS website (overcomingms.org) is a great way to learn about the wide world of possibilities with this Program and the group of wise and dedicated people who have developed and disseminated it. The website can help with new cooking techniques and tasty recipes, general lifestyle information and inspirational stories of how people with MS manage MS.

Staying motivated and engaged with the OMS philosophy for the long haul is vitally important to sustain commitment to all the aspects of the OMS Program. Doing so with a positive, active and conscious mindset will help you to continuously improve yourself, maintain independence and above all enjoy the adventure of transforming your health.

MS is a disorder that is very poorly understood by the community, not to mention many in the medical profession. I was often asked by people who knew my diagnosis when I was first diagnosed if it was contagious. This unnecessary fear could really harm close personal friendships and I had to be very cautious about who I disclosed to. I was and am very open to discussing MS, but it is a complex condition that cannot be easily explained in a few short sentences. It was quite difficult not to start giving a long lecture about what MS is, who gets it and why, especially to casual acquaintances, so I often found it was easier not to bring the subject up if they didn't know me well. Irish lawyer Gregory Hendron gives specific advice about disclosure in Chapter 15.

Clear communication with close family members, particularly blood relatives, remains vital to not only assist you on your MS path but also to educate them about how they can help reduce the likelihood of developing MS themselves. As a positive side effect, overall improvement in their general physical and mental health is a likely consequence.

In summary, the OMS road to recovery is backed by powerful and compelling scientific evidence. The Program also provides a life-changing promise of hope, which is what we crave when coping with the challenges of managing this complex, often frightening and unpredictable condition.

Ground covered

The OMS Program is a comprehensive suite of lifestyle modifications that, when combined together and integrated into a daily routine, have been shown to reduce the impact of MS. In many people the OMS lifestyle approach can stop or greatly reduce episodes or attacks and reverse some symptoms and adverse effects, although these changes may take some time to fully evolve.

OMS is a sound, scientifically based and researched program, the elements of which have been slowly accepted by a sceptical medical establishment. For many decades the Swank regimen, which has some similar aspects to the OMS Program, has generally not been embraced by neurologists. However, the participants who followed the regimen carefully lived long and healthy lives not limited by their MS. Recent research has verified the value of the primary elements of the Swank program, especially the need to reduce as much saturated fat in the diet as possible. The OMS Program has refined the dietary principles and introduced other changes to further enhance the beneficial effects.

OMS is a self-directed and strongly empowering strategy to improve wellness. Having the tools and knowledge of what we can do for ourselves gives us the hope and the strength to take control of a frightening and often bewildering condition. We can actively work towards and look forward to a better future rather than be burdened by the dismal prospects we faced when first diagnosed.

The OMS Program can not only improve the course of MS but also has the added bonus of counteracting many of the health problems that are a result of our Western lifestyle. The combination of a low-saturated-fat diet, optimal omega-3 and vitamin D levels, exercise, de-stressing and social inclusion can improve mental and physical wellness for anyone, especially those of us dealing with a chronic disease.

My Story: Phil King

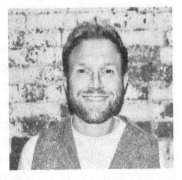

I was diagnosed with MS following a bout of optic neuritis in October 2012. Hot on the heels of the optic neuritis came several, previously unknown symptoms: unusual sensations in both of my legs, as if they were unable to carry me; burning all over my body very similar to acute sunburn; dizzi-ness, fatigue and deafness; and strange numbness, particularly in my fingers. I felt very scared as I had always been highly fit and active. I didn't want my wife Lizzie or my children Laurence and Lottie to become my caregivers.

I was lucky as I had heard about the book *Overcoming Multiple Sclerosis* by Professor George Jelinek just before I was diagnosed. I immediately ordered the book and read it cover to cover.

I found the program proposed by the book very compelling and straight to the point. I switched very quickly to a wholefood diet sup-plemented with seafood; I knew I had to 'dump the junk'. I had always enjoyed seafood so that wasn't a problem. I was so desperate for good health that a diet rich in nutrients didn't seem like an effort.

I had started running for exercise many years ago as an aid to stopping smoking; running had become another addiction for me and one that I wasn't going to relinquish easily. To read that running in sunshine could be beneficial for the production of vitamin D was an added benefit; however, getting lots of sun exposure in England can prove difficult so I also supplement daily with vitamin D3.

I have always been a person who can become easily anxious. In other words, I worry a lot! I downloaded albums by Deepak Chopra and Professor Mark Williams (from Oxford University) onto Spotify and these have helped my mindfulness journey a great deal.

I was determined that all this change would be for life. I wasn't going to let the odd unhealthy snack anywhere near my program, or occasionally skip my meditation—I wanted to remain as healthy as I could possibly be.

I decided that I didn't want to take any disease-modifying medications. This was my own personal choice. I took the view that if after a year of following the OMS Program I deteriorated further, I would then review my decision.

I have been following the OMS principles for eight years now and I am happy to report that I have not relapsed in all this time. I get occasional 'ghosts of symptoms past' but nothing more than that. I exercise six days a week, either running a 6-mile circuit or doing weight training. I am fitter now than I was before I was diagnosed with MS. The disease doesn't worry me anymore and I feel that my overall outlook is good. I have now become an MS nurse in a bid to help others diagnosed with MS. My good health is all thanks to the OMS Program. I am eternally grateful.

3

Eat well

Jack McNulty

> Changing to the OMS diet was a challenge at first,
> but is now a joy; I wouldn't eat any other way.
>
> Karen Costello-McFeat, Eastbourne, UK, OMSer,
> chef and food instructor

Diet as part of the OMS lifestyle

The dietary part of the OMS lifestyle is possibly the most discussed (even debated) element of the entire OMS Program. In fact, I often see others referring to the Program simply as the 'OMS Diet' even though diet represents a single element within a broader lifestyle plan. Describing the entire Program as a diet also implies a temporary state of affairs—sort of like a weight-loss program. But this is far from the intention of the Program. All of the elements are meant as permanent lifelong changes in lifestyle and dietary behaviour—a daunting prospect for many.

I believe the dietary guidelines generate much discussion and debate because there are so many moving parts to consider. It is not as simple as selecting A or B as with other components of the Program. You are either exercising or you're not . . . you are either taking vitamin D or you're not . . . you are either meditating or you're not. With diet there are cultural considerations that determine what different people eat; there are social pressures from friends, family and co-workers that may influence dietary choices; there are economic issues to take into account; access to certain products is not the same worldwide; cooking knowledge differs widely; there are work–life balance issues to consider; even physical limitations enter into daily dietary decisions— things like fatigue, disability, cognitive decline, and the senses taste and smell. All of these factors need proper

Changing one's diet is more complex than other parts of the OMS Program and is influenced by many factors

consideration by the person with MS at least 2–4 times per day— every day!

No wonder it is tempting for some to turn to the ocean of dietary information and opinions polluting the internet to answer their questions, justify maintaining their current behaviour or look for that elusive quick fix. This path often leads to further confusion or misinterpretation of facts—and that is a dangerous gamble when health is on the line.

This chapter covers the OMS diet in simple, factual terms, covering broader guidelines of the diet, the variances permitted and common issues that most people need to address. The goal is to encourage those who are looking to jump onto the road to recovery and inspire current program adherents to remain on that road. This is not a comprehensive look at all the details concerning what to eat and what not to eat. Those facts, and many more, have been covered in earlier publications. Updated information can be found on the Overcoming Multiple Sclerosis website (overcomingms.org). You can review evidence-based diet information by reading the *Overcoming Multiple Sclerosis* book. You can also pick up valuable cooking tips and ideas from the OMS cookbook. Information about obtaining these books can be found on the OMS website.

Getting all the information is the simple part. Dealing with the 'how' issues—the specifics on how to navigate the diet based on most individual circumstances—is where you will encounter the challenges. This is where the rubber meets the road as the journey begins.

What is the goal of the OMS Program?

Most of us begin the OMS diet with a certain degree of trep-idation. I can imagine how challenging it is for someone newly diagnosed, who is already filled with anxiety, to read the guide-lines and think about the potential disruptions to their life that wait just around the corner. When viewed from this perspective, only restrictions come into focus and it is difficult for some to see anything other than all those details. Dietary limitations might even be magnified when we carefully consider the real-life impact the diet has on our current eating, cooking, shopping and social habits. For most of us, there is a good chance we will need to sig-nificantly modify our dietary habits before beginning the journey on this road to good health.

Like confronting any overwhelming task, I think it can be helpful to take a moment and step back to gain a broader per-spective. Ask yourself a simple question—a question you can ask at the beginning of the journey or at any other point along the way. What is your main objective? I'm betting most people want to get back some degree of normality in their life. To create the best possible chance of minimising the risk of MS progression—perhaps even allow some space to think about recovery. To put it another way, most of us want to maintain or improve our overall quality of life.

Great—this is exactly the goal of the OMS Program. In fact, a large number of studies now show that MS is a lifestyle disease, which means that if we can make some important life-style changes, we will greatly improve our chances of meeting this ultimate objective.

Here's another fact. If we can influence the overall chemical make-up of our blood (what I will call the blood profile) each time we eat something, then we will nudge even closer to meeting our ultimate objective. This means we need to do what we can to change the profile of fats within our blood. We need to shift from the abundance of saturated fats common in a Western diet towards a greater proportion of healthier, polyunsaturated fats, also known as omega-6 and omega-3 fatty acids. Saturated fats tend to be 'sticky', encouraging clotting and other abnormal processes, while unsaturated fats tend to be less sticky and more fluid, and have healthier properties. Dramatically reducing saturated fat intake minimises cell degeneration.

We also need to alter the ratio of the polyunsaturated fats, decreasing intake of omega-6 and increasing intake of omega-3 fatty acids, to reduce inflammation markers.

We need to eat a diet rich in fibre and remain properly hydrated to lessen the impact of chronic conditions like fatigue. The scientific studies are clear about all of these dietary impacts. These steps lead to a more favourable blood profile—one that helps the body slow MS progression and even reverse symptoms in some people.

To be clear, changing lifelong habits is not simple. But understanding your goals and seeing how they align with OMS objectives will help you navigate the challenging curves and ever-changing peaks and valleys that await you. The first step is to get on the road and decide which lane to drive in. And most importantly, you must understand the importance of staying within the guardrails that protect you from driving off the road.

The best route to a healthy diet

Everything you eat can represent an opportunity to improve your overall blood profile and your life!

That's a remarkable statement. Think about it. We have the ultimate control over what we eat and how we nourish our bodies, yet most of us forget this one basic fact and relinquish control to someone else—a restaurant, a mega-corporation, the latest trends and fads on the internet, and so on. In order for us to retain our control, we must remain focused on what outcome we want. To put it another way, we must focus on how we can stay on the road to good health and allow enough room for our own unique life situation.

Let's stick with this road metaphor a bit longer to help us understand how to navigate this tricky condition more safely. Imagine that you are driving on a highway with a number of lanes. This is your road to recovery; the guardrails on each side represent the barriers. These are the limitations of your new dietary lifestyle. The lanes allow you to drive at different speeds, and it's perfectly acceptable to move from one lane to another as often as you wish. These lanes represent the slight differences people make within the dietary guidelines to help them live more happily or to treat some other kind of underlying health issue.

Let's use gluten as an example. Some decide to include gluten as part of their diet, while others resolve to greatly reduce gluten or even eliminate it from their diet. In each case, gluten represents a different lane, but it's still acceptable within the overall guidelines and you haven't left the road in either case. The use of oil in cooking is another example—one that is often debated. Healthy oils are allowed on this highway, but if you're choosing to drive in that lane, then you need to be aware of a few potential potholes that can cause you to suddenly veer off the road (more on the topic of fats will come later in this chapter).

The science is clear—influencing and improving our blood profile through the foods we consume can help maintain or improve overall quality of life

~

Most of us already know that many doctors and scientists agree on the healthiest diet to prevent and treat most diseases: a whole-food, plant-based (WFPB) diet. On its own, this diet will greatly reduce saturated fat intake, consumption of inflammation-inducing foods, and chemicals subsequently produced in the body called free radicals that cause cell degeneration, as well as improve overall gut health through increased fibre and vegetables.

But there are many factors to consider when trying to define this kind of diet in real and practical terms. For instance, you could choose a restrictive, WFPB diet encouraged by some health experts that eliminates all oils in cooking and does not allow for nuts or high-fat wholefoods like avocados. Another group of doctors encourages the same diet, but allows for nuts and avocados to be consumed in moderate amounts. A third group takes the same elements and stipulates it is okay to consume 'healthy' expelled oils. The OMS Program is considered as a fourth option. It allows for 'healthy' fish consumption in addition to the same guidelines as the third dietary group.

All of these options represent the entire road to good health, and each option can be viewed as a separate lane. You should consider getting on it as soon as possible after your diagnosis. You get to decide which lane to drive in based on your personal needs and situation—and it's perfectly okay to move from one lane to another whenever your situation changes.

Now let's take a closer look at the different lanes and understand the potential hazards that may cause some difficulties—especially significant when just beginning the journey.

The first lane—the one that limits the diet to whole, plant-based foods without nuts and avocados—is the most difficult to drive in right from the start. Not only are food choices limited under this diet, but the cooking methods might also be unfamiliar to some. Choices when eating in restaurants could be severely restricted, leading to potential conflicts with friends and family (restaurant food is discussed in more detail later in this chapter, but make a note now that most restaurant food is a flashing yellow light warning). Although this diet is great in reducing fat consumption, a problem may occur if you also restrict your overall essential fatty acid intake—especially the immune-modulating omega-3 fatty acids. It is also possible that fat intake is too low to absorb enough critical fat-soluble vitamins. This is a great lane for those who are experienced—or perhaps even for part-time visitors. It requires a good understanding of all nutritional implications (it may be a good idea to work with a licensed dietician), good working knowledge on how to shop for food and cook it, and a strong social support network.

The second lane includes nuts and high-fat wholefoods like avocados and offers more food choices (it's amazing what can be done with nuts these days) and a slightly higher fat intake. The risk of not consuming enough fats in this lane is reduced—in fact, the opposite is true. One common problem for those electing to start in this lane is eating too many nuts and avocados. They are great fillers for quick snacks, and they are versatile in the kitchen (for those in the know, nut-based vegan cheeses are relatively simple to make, as is an avocado-based chocolate mousse). But even though these foods are tasty additions to the diet, there is a risk of eating too much and taking in too many inflammation-producing fats. This is another great lane to travel in for those who are relatively experienced and possess good knowledge of nutritional requirements, cooking techniques and a strong social support network. Most experienced OMS Program participants spend a good deal of their time in this lane.

The third lane allows for the inclusion of 'healthy' expelled oils, meaning unrefined oils squeezed or expelled from foods such as fruits, olives, nuts, seeds and grains. The choices of what you can eat increase, but the cooking methods can be challenging as they require an understanding of oil chemistry and that warning light just started to flash a bit brighter. The term 'healthy expelled oils' may seem simple enough to understand, but trust me, it is far from clear. Deciding to include oils in your food and cooking is an individual choice, so let's take a moment to understand some of the issues that could cause problems (more detail will follow in this chapter).

A healthy oil is an oil that is not refined or already oxidised. But how do you make this determination as a consumer? Then there is the balance of fats within the oil to consider—is it primarily polyunsaturated or monounsaturated? (Remember, stay away from oils that are primarily saturated.) The use of the term 'cold pressed' is unregulated worldwide and manufacturers have used it to imply a healthy oil, even though it is usually not. Cold pressing also explains nothing about what happens to that oil after pressing. It could be heated to extreme temperatures and chemically deodorised to create shelf-life stability and longevity. This is a refined oil. It is also impossible to know how the oil is treated once it enters the supply chain and sits on supermarket shelves or in a warehouse. The same can be said for marketing terms like 'extra virgin'. There are no standards worldwide for the use of this term that imply some kind of healthy oil (except for European Union guidelines governing extra virgin olive oil). I will go into more detail on fats in the next section, but for now, let me state that this lane offers a broader selection of foods, with some increased risks. You should invest a good amount of time to investigate oil choices wherever you are in the world.

The fourth lane is the lane most people begin in because it represents the simplest transition by including fish. Oily fish are an excellent source of valuable omega-3 essential fatty acids, but they also have higher amounts of saturated fats and should be consumed in moderation. Seafood (like calamari, mussels, octopus, clams, and so on) have relatively small amounts of fats, and that makes these foods attractive for some—especially when eating out or while on holiday. Fish, however, present a few additional obstacles to consider. The amount of toxic pollution in the waters where fish live is a significant issue to consider, and perhaps a strong enough reason to consider limiting overall intake. Microplastic contamination is another reason to limit fish in the diet.

The OMS diet is flexible and has many potential variations but it is wise not to compromise the broad guidelines

Keeping your dietary decisions within the broad guidelines outlined above is your on-ramp. Choosing which lane works best for you is a personal decision based on your current life situation. These guidelines may help you achieve your health goals by preventing cell degeneration, reducing overall inflammation in the body and improving gut health to help address common ailments.

Congratulations—you are now on the road to recovery. Now, let's figure out how to drive safely by looking closely at some of the potential hazards that lie ahead. We will begin with fats, move

to cooking methods and finish with 'rest stops and off-ramps'—
the flexibility that you can exercise when shopping, travelling and
social dining.

Managing fats in your diet

Many doctors and scientific studies hold that diets high in fat
lead to degenerative diseases like MS. But what they really mean
is diets high in saturated fat. This apparent conflict gets to the
heart of perhaps the most debated part of the OMS diet—how
to manage fat intake and whether to include oils in our cooking.
Let's explore these questions in greater detail.

Fats and oils are a complicated nutritional topic. There is
a great deal of information already published concerning fat-
intake amounts and the type of fats that we should be including
in our diet. You can refer to the *Overcoming Multiple Sclerosis*
book or the OMS website to find the latest scientific information
on fats and oils as they apply to our lifestyle. Another excellent
resource to check out is Udo Erasmus's book *Fats That Heal, Fats
That Kill*. These excellent resources will help you understand how
to navigate this topic with more security and confidence.

As stated earlier, the OMS nutritional approach includes the
use of oils. In fact, the HOLISM study
indicates that people with MS who
regularly consume flaxseed oil have
60 per cent fewer relapses than those
who don't, after accounting for other
lifestyle factors. We also know that
the human body needs some fats for
survival. These 'essential fatty acids'
are critical in our diet, but this does not
mean that we need to ingest oils to get
enough of these fats, because we can
get them from food sources. So why
include any oil in our cooking at all?

Most oil use in recipes is purely for enjoyment, but it remains important to consume adequate amounts of omega-3 fatty acids through natural food sources or oil supplementation or both

The importance of fat intake was
not well known until the early 1900s,

when scientists began to identify essential fatty acids and critical fat-soluble vitamins. Over the last century, crops and diets have changed in most developed countries, such that omega-3 essential fatty acids are now present and consumed in very low amounts, particularly for people avoiding seafood. But mostly, adding oils is for human pleasure. Fats and oils add moisture, improve flavour and change the texture of our food. That's it. Once you understand these roles, it is much easier to decide whether using oils in our cooking is appropriate, even on a recipe-by-recipe basis.

Fats (including all oils) are mostly perceived as a sweet taste sensation. They can leave a velvety smooth coating in our mouth to which we have grown accustomed from diets relatively high in processed foods. Basically, we have become addicted to the flavour and sensation of fats/oils. Fortunately, we can easily wean ourselves off this reliance by drastically reducing overall fat intake for a few weeks. Long-time OMS dieters usually report experiencing a renewed sense of taste and flavours that were previously hidden by an overabundance of fats in their diet.

Fats and oils play a significant role in changing the texture of our food. Because fats/oils are highly effective in heat transfer, they are often used to speed the caramelising of sugars or the browning of proteins to create flavourful outer crusts on foods. Fats/oils also act as an effective emulsifier when mixing liquids and proteins to create a creamy sensation—think mayonnaise or ice cream as examples of this function.

Fats/oils also work to limit the structure of gluten networks when water and flour are mixed together. Mixtures containing high amounts of fat will have shorter gluten strands and a fluffy, cake-like structure (this is why fats are also called shortenings—they literally shorten the gluten network). Shortbread and crumbly cakes are excellent examples of this effect, while oil-free breads like baguettes tend to have a much leaner interior structure.

Fats and oils help food retain the natural moisture content of food during cooking by limiting evaporation. Vegetables roasted in the oven or sautéed on the stove without any fat/oil often taste drier than those roasted with fats/oils. Baked goods such as cakes suffer the same fate without any added fats/oils.

Fortunately, much of the impact to moisture content can be compensated for by adding a liquid to the food or by adding something like a fruit puree to baked goods. Compensating for the lack of fats/oils by using substitutes does not easily achieve flaky textures (in cakes, for example). You will need to either use a fat/oil in your recipe to create flakiness or get used to a less flaky texture. Using starches instead of fat to emulsify proteins and liquid is possible and effective, so even delicious preparations like lemon curd are possible on the OMS diet.

Let's return briefly to our road metaphor. You will recall healthy expelled oils are encouraged on the OMS Program. But it is also clear that the majority of food we cook can be prepared without the addition of any oil. Your main consideration in deciding whether or not to use oil in your cooking comes down to a question of pleasure but can also be one of need if not consuming enough omega-3 essential fatty acids.

Which oils to use in cooking?

Many people following the OMS diet make a personal decision to use oils in their cooking from time to time—especially in baking. Choosing the right oil to use is the first challenge. Once you've made your purchase, it is important to understand how to prevent the oil from oxidising too quickly. Preventing further degradation of the oil during the cooking process is also important to limit harmful substances forming.

All oils share certain characteristics. They all have some poly-unsaturated omega-3 and omega-6, monounsaturated omega-9 and saturated fats—but in differing ratios. The guidelines we are following on the OMS Program instruct us to strive for a ratio of omega-3 to omega-6 fatty acids of around 3:1 so we can keep our inflammation markers as low as possible. Most of us develop a certain degree of awareness about how to track this intake, so no measuring is necessary. New participants in the OMS Program should develop a good understanding of the fat ratios in the foods and oils they consume. The OMS website is an excellent resource to turn to for more information on this topic. It is important to be aware that most foods have considerably more omega-6 than 3 and therefore we suggest supplementing with omega-3 oils.

We also need to consider how oils can become harmful. All oils slowly break down and become rancid. Exposure to heat, light and air over a period of time causes oils to oxidise and develop stale, cardboard-like aromas with hints of old paint and harsh, bitter flavours. This doesn't even sound good, and for good reason. Oils with these characteristics are rancid—they are not safe to consume. Let's look at each of these negative effects separately and discover how we can minimise them.

Purchasing the freshest possible oil is your first priority. In some parts of the world, it is possible to get the oils fresh from the supplier soon after production and packaging. It is helpful to look for dates on the bottle whenever possible. As an example, extra virgin olive oils in Europe must contain an expiration date on the bottle—it is 18 months after bottling. Most oils don't have a date on the bottle, so it may be wise to contact the producer of the oil or ask the store manager.

Oils should be stored in a cool, dark place. Refrigerating oils with high amounts of omega-3 fatty acids is mandatory. It is not necessary to refrigerate other oils, but it is also not harmful to the oil if you have the space. Freezing oils is also effective in slowing down the oxidation rate. Many OMS Program followers tend to purchase flaxseed oil in bulk and simply freeze it until needed. Oils begin to oxidise immediately when exposed to air and light. Oils that are primarily omega-3 (flax, hemp, walnut, pumpkin) deteriorate the fastest—usually within 6–9 weeks. They begin to taste bitter and should be discarded. Consumed rancid oils generate free radicals within the body; over time these

Fresh oils should be expelled properly, with minimal processing, and be properly stored; pay careful attention to protecting oil during cooking

free radicals damage cells and cause degeneration. Oils that are mostly omega-6 (sunflower, rapeseed, sesame) fully oxidise in 3–6 months. Monounsaturated oils (extra virgin olive oil) should last for 12–18 months.

Applying heat to oil speeds the rate of deterioration, so fresh oils perform better than oils that have partially oxidised. But that's not the only consideration. All oils begin to rapidly degrade at a temperature of 120° C (248° F). Frying with oil raises the temperature much higher, releasing what are called frying breakdown products. These chemicals are especially toxic when consumed. Even at lower temperatures, when an oil reaches a temperature where it begins to emit gasses, it has reached its 'smoke point'. Not only are the smoky fumes noxious, but the residual fatty acids remaining in the pan or pot become harmful to consume, and ruin the flavour of the food anyway. Smoke points for oils vary depending on a number of factors—most notably their unsaturated fatty acid content: the higher the unsaturated fatty acid content, the more unstable the fat and the lower the smoke point. Smoke points on labels or in marketing material don't really tell us much. It's much better to limit heat exposure as much as possible during the cooking process.

We will discuss various cooking methods and how heat is transferred to food in the next section. For now, we'll focus on some simple strategies to help control oil temperatures during the cooking process. Let's begin with liquid. The boiling point of liquids is mostly fixed at a temperature far below the point when oils begin to degrade. This means we can put oil into boiling water and it will be relatively safe for an extended period of time. It also implies that we don't actually need the pot of water to keep the oil safe with other cooking methods, because the same rule applies across the board: water prevents oils from reaching temperatures above the water's boiling point. This is why it is perfectly fine to add a bit of oil to sautéed onions in a frypan along with a spoonful of water (it's even better to add the oil to the onions at the end of the cooking process). This fact also means that it is safe to roast vegetables in a hot oven with a light coating of oil and a spoonful or two of water in the pan. Steam and pressure also control temperatures: steam is the same as boiling water, and pressure applied to cooking raises boiling points by about 20 per cent—still below the threshold of 120°C (248°F)—the point where oils begin to degrade.

Using fresh, healthy expelled oils is perfectly fine within the OMS dietary guidelines. But is it important to purchase fresh oils, store them correctly and then apply some simple strategies to control heat exposure during the cooking process. Following these simple steps reduces the likelihood of elevated exposure to factors leading to cell degeneration and increased inflammation.

Healthy cooking methods

Cooking can be described in simple terms as using heat to prepare food for human consumption. This is a very important concept to understand when trying to cook healthy foods.

To begin understanding how heat works in cooking, we need to first establish an important fact—cooking temperatures do not directly correlate to food temperature. Here's what I mean. We all know water boils at a temperature close to 100°C (212°F) and it would instantly hurt to put your finger in that boiling pot of water. On the other hand, you can set your oven temperature to 100°C (212°F) and stick your entire arm in the oven for several minutes without it hurting. The difference is due to how heat is transferred from the source to whatever is being heated.

In the first example, water is heated when the heat source (the burner) transfers heat to the pot, which heats the water inside. The water now becomes the heat source that cooks something— such as potatoes or beans. The temperature never rises above the boiling point in this example. So the heat remains relatively low, but the transfer of heat is fast. (Can you still feel that finger you put into the water?)

The heat source in the second example is the radiating coils at the top and bottom of the oven. They are heated to the temperature that is set—in our example it is 100°C (212°F). The heat source transfers to the air in the oven, which now heats anything placed in the oven as well as radiating off the oven walls. Obviously, the space inside the oven and a circulating fan dictate how fast the air will heat to the desired temperature. Anything placed inside the oven will instantly cool the air temperature (opening the oven door will cause the inside air temperature to drop by 25 per cent within a half-minute) and require a significant amount of time to heat whatever is being cooked. The larger the item, the longer it will take for the heat to penetrate the core.

Let's take it a step further and discuss how heat is transferred in every cooking method to fully grasp what this implies for cooking under the OMS Program.

Moist heat transfers energy (heat) through water and steam. It is highly efficient and works rapidly. Moist heat cooking involves these methods: boiling, steaming, poaching, braising or stewing. The maximum temperature in these cooking methods is 100°C (212°F). Pressure cooking is a type of moist heat because it relies on a change of pressure to heat small amounts of water rapidly. The difference in pressure means the maximum temperature of the liquid rises to 120°C (248°F). Microwave cooking is also considered a type of moist heat cooking because the heat source (the microwaves) are applied to moisture, which transfers to whatever is being cooked. One major difference with microwave cooking is that the heat is applied from the inside of whatever is being cooked and moves to the surface.

Dry heat cooking methods transfer heat either directly or indirectly. Think of the difference between putting something directly on a heat source and placing it inside an oven as previously discussed.

Food temperatures can be tempered and controlled by moist cooking techniques or using indirect heat-transfer methods

The direct method of cooking includes sautéing, frying and grilling over an open flame. This method of cooking rapidly raises the temperature of whatever is being cooked. The indirect method of cooking includes baking and roasting. This method constrains cooking temperatures and the food takes longer to reach a set temperature.

Let's investigate a couple of examples to see how these concepts play out in the OMS kitchen.

Sautéing is a common method of cooking. In a classical cooking sense, a cook will quickly cook smaller pieces of food in a small amount of fat over high heat. Here's what that means in terms of transferring heat to the food. The pan is placed directly on a burner and heated to a temperature between 180°C (350°F) and 220°C (428°F). Once the pan becomes quite hot, fat is added to the hot pan and the food goes into the pan and the hot fat. Obviously the food will cook quickly in this environment, and so will the fat. And if you recall our previous discussion about fats and temperature, the fats in the pan begin breaking down at around 120°C (248°F)—or very shortly after the fat enters the pan. Assuming nothing else is added to the pan, the temperature of the fat that the food is cooking in will easily reach unhealthy levels and begin to create harmful elements in the food. This is why this method of cooking is not recommended.

Cooking foods in a small amount of liquid in a frypan on the stove is often referred to as water-sautéing. In reality, this is a moist heat cooking method rather than a dry heat method that is commonly associated with sautéing. But the name doesn't really matter. What's important to understand is how the water works to cool the food temperature. And because it is impossible for water to reach temperatures above boiling point, whatever we are cooking will not reach temperatures above boiling point—a crucial fact to consider when deciding whether you want to add any oil to your food.

Let's take a look at what happens to temperatures when we bake a loaf of bread. A medium-sized loaf of bread is best when baked at a high temperature—something around 230°C (450°F). This high temperature in the oven is important because we want the bread to bake within 30–40 minutes—the time it will take for the heat to penetrate to the core and cook the starches and proteins, giving the bread its structure. The surface of the bread heats at a faster rate than the interior. The sugars in the starch begin to caramelise and the proteins denature—this gives the bread a crust. Interestingly, the surface of the bread only has enough time to reach about 130°C (265°F) and the interior of the bread never goes above 95°C (203°F). The implications are clear if we add oil to the bread—the temperature of the oil remains in the safe zone (less than 120°C (248°F). This same principle can be applied to other baked items such as cakes, and what this means is simple—it is okay to bake items at higher temperatures because cooking temperatures do not directly correlate to the food temperature.

Excessive heat in cooking can create harmful elements in the foods we eat. The result is increased cell degeneration and elevated inflammatory markers in our blood profile. We have already discussed the problems that occur when we expose oils to temperatures above 120°C (248°F). Excessive heat applied to carbohydrates and proteins may also create problems. Science is just beginning to understand these issues in more detail, but we all know it's not a good idea to eat too much charred toast.

Rest stops and off-ramps

Like any long journey, there are times when you need to stop and take a rest. So what would that look like when you're driving on the road to good health?

Let's take a peek at a striking revelation regarding this exact topic made by Dr Swank in his book *The Multiple Sclerosis Diet Book*. To paraphrase his findings, Dr Swank discovered that most so-called bad dieters (those that came off his program—even for a short period) suffered more relapses once they moved away from the guidelines. This flashing red warning light made a lasting impression on me, and continues to guide my daily dietary decisions—as it should with anyone following the OMS diet. There are no exits on this road to good health, but there are situations that come up from time to time that demand a certain degree of flexibility.

You are not expected to cook every meal using only organic wholefoods from a farm 2 kilometres away. As nice as that sounds, it is also completely unrealistic and impossible to achieve. This means that there will be times when you will want to dine in a restaurant—and probably with friends or family who may not follow the same strict guidelines you're following. What do you do?

Most restaurant food is not compliant with the guidelines that I have laid out in this chapter. Sadly, that's just the reality these days. Many restaurants—especially chain restaurants—do not even have a large kitchen because their food is prepared off-site in a central kitchen. This is the trend in the restaurant business in order to cut back on costs, and it will only become more prevalent going forward. This also means that almost everyone working in these restaurants has no idea how a menu item is prepared and exactly what ingredients were used.

Stay within the broad OMS dietary guidelines; however, unintentional mistakes and compromising situations are of course inevitable—they are learning opportunities

Here's a simple example of how that might affect you—even with simple items like bread. Bread is rarely prepared in a restaurant. It is purchased from a local bakery and delivered to the restaurant. There will be a document in the restaurant that will list the ingredients, so this is handy when you ask what's in the bread. But it's not always clear what E472 is as an ingredient, and now you are uncomfortable—do you eat the bread or leave it alone? Avoiding the bread, you decide to have something safe like spaghetti with tomato sauce. Okay, that sounds fine, but do you really know what kind of oil they used to prepare that tomato sauce? Do you know if the oil was heated too much . . . and for too long?

It is impractical to limit your dining to what you would do in your own kitchen. Whenever you step outside and dine elsewhere, you are relinquishing control over the ingredients and methods used to cook the food you are ordering. For the most part, this is perfectly fine, but you can minimise the impact. Try to call ahead to the restaurant you are planning to visit. Speak with the chef directly, if possible, and ask about options that would fit your requirements. This strategy works especially well with restaurants that have small menus, and that brings me to the next tip. Any restaurant that has a large menu will be inflexible. Most of the food is pre-made and only warmed at the time of ordering. Large and crowded restaurants also tend to be inflexible. Kitchens are busy places. Even if you pre-arranged something special with the kitchen, a busy cook will not necessarily follow those instructions (I know—I've been on that side of a restaurant). Chain restaurants tend to be the most inflexible and work off a business model that is geared towards low cost and high revenue. This means ingredients used in chain restaurants will be the lowest cost items available. Can you imagine the quality of oils used in these restaurants?

Oh, remember that E472 ingredient listed in the bread example? That's a common emulsifier and leavening agent used in many commercial breads. It is generally considered safe for human consumption, which doesn't exactly fill me with confidence. But it is also important to put things in perspective. The amounts of whatever you ingest will be so low that they will not have an impact, unless of course you make it a habit and eat this way on a regular basis. This is a gentle way of saying it is probably best to make your own food from ingredients that you purchase and understand, and keep restaurant dining to a moderate to limited level. And if you find yourself in this situation, enjoy the food in a mindful manner, then make sure you spend a few days driving in lane number one—the lane that emphasises a WFPB diet, with no added oils, nuts or avocados, in order to compensate.

Understand your unique dietary needs and what works best for you, allowing room for flexibility, but without compromising on broader guidelines

Remember, the OMS diet is a single part of a broader lifestyle program. Mastering it is important, but take care not to micromanage the details (especially if you are just starting out). Some people enjoy getting involved with all the details, but for most this could lead to increased stress and reverse many of the benefits you're trying to achieve with the diet.

Stay within the guardrails, decide which lane works for you—but also allow yourself the freedom to change lanes and manage a particular situation. And don't forget to just stay on the road!

Ground covered

Managing the dietary component of the OMS Program is more complex than other parts of the self-management program. There are many individual factors that come into play: social, cultural, financial, physical, to name a few. Fortunately, there is a great deal of flexibility within the broader guidelines of the diet to help the vast majority of people navigate it successfully.

The dietary guidelines outlined in the OMS Program are a single element of the Program. Incorporating the diet can greatly effect positive change in most people by influencing and improving blood profile through the foods consumed on a daily basis.

Most studies agree that diets high in saturated and human-made fats lead to degenerative diseases. Use of oils in OMS-safe recipes is optional; however, it is critical to consume adequate amounts of omega-3 essential fatty acids. If one chooses to use oils, then special attention and care must be given to purchasing healthy and fresh oils that are primarily unsaturated, storing them correctly and using correct cooking methods to control oil degradation during the cooking process. It is also critical to ensure that the diet is rich in fibre and antioxidants from a wide variety of plants to ensure a favourable blood profile.

Even though the broader OMS dietary guidelines are fixed, most people eventually make unintentional mistakes or encounter compromising situations that fall outside the OMS recommendations. These issues alone have minimal overall impact on a person's health as long as they are not consistently made or viewed as an occasional reward or treat. Ultimately, the OMS Program allows for a great deal of flexibility and room to meet unique social, cultural, financial and physical needs.

My Story: Ingrid Adelsberger

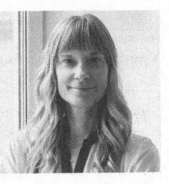

I was diagnosed with MS in 2011 and didn't have any limitations for about eight years. I had some symptoms but they were so mild that I didn't think much about them. Then I had my wonderful daughter. Since then my symptoms have been stronger (she is 23 months old at the time of writing). I realised that during pregnancy and the first six months of my daughter's life, I didn't eat too well and certainly did not meditate or exercise enough.

Today I am better but I had some difficult phases during the last year and a half and I am not yet where I want to be. Maybe some symptoms are new; mostly they are not and only partly stronger.

I have learned so much on this journey. Since the beginning I have focused on food and that is why I wanted to write the *Overcoming Multiple Sclerosis Cookbook* because I learned that I was not the only one wanting to eat good food while on the OMS diet. I think counting saturated fat is easy so that is why I focused on it. Today I think differently about food and how to eat healthier: nutrition for me is about a lot more than just counting fats. I think the balance is what is important. For example, I often make macro bowls with vegetables, tofu, beans and grains and a salad on the side, all covered with an interesting OMS-friendly sauce that turns a bland meal into a tasty one.

I move as much as I can daily. I try not to think of it as exercise. Being a health coach, I have worked with a lot of people who dislike the word 'exercise' so I embrace any movement. Some days it is just running errands, using stairs and walking a lot! Sometimes I have time for additional workouts.

I meditate daily. It has taken me years, plus a lot of fear around going through these difficult phases, to build a consistent meditation practice. I also believe that meditation has helped me to get through the rough patches and helps me to keep my mood positive.

I like guided meditations because of the prompts and the positive mindset of the meditation teacher.

When people say that with MS you only get worse, it makes me sad. I hope I can show them a new picture of MS (because we know many in the OMS community who remain the same or got better!). I do not want to pressure myself or fail them in the picture that I want them to see. That again is a huge lesson because it is about me and not them.

I am positive, though, that I can get to my pre-pregnancy baseline where I had almost no symptoms. I have a good quality of life now but I want to have a better one, like I had before. I try to focus on what I can versus what I cannot do (and sometimes that is hard). With rest, I can do mostly everything. I want to be a mum and wife who can do (almost) everything with my family. It is easy to be motivated by my wonderful daughter and amazing husband.

4

Get enough sun and vitamin D

Dr Conor Kerley

Thanks to the OMS Program I am living; my life is transformed, for which I am eternally grateful.

Alison Marwick, Surrey, UK

There are many things to consider when looking at the relationship between sun and vitamin D and MS, in terms of how they affect the risk of getting MS in the first place and how they affect the progression of the disease. Sunlight acts on the skin to produce vitamin D, which in turn affects MS risk and progression, but sunlight also has a direct effect in its own right. These effects will be considered in turn, but firstly, let's look more closely at what vitamin D is, how it is formed and how it affects health.

As an individual nutrient, vitamin D has probably gained the most attention in the MS field. The highest level of evidence about any medical intervention is the randomised controlled trial (RCT), or preferably a synthesis (meta-analysis) of several randomised controlled trials. RCTs are where researchers randomly allocate trial participants to the treatment being studied or an inactive placebo. Surprisingly, there are no substantial randomised controlled trials on the role of vitamin D in MS. But there is a wealth of other scientific evidence showing that vitamin D is important for preventing MS and for keeping people with MS healthy. To a lesser extent there is similar evidence for sun exposure in its own right.

What is vitamin D?

Vitamin D, like all vitamins, is essential for life in humans. However, vitamin D has many features that make it unique compared with other vitamins. Vitamin D is more accurately described as a pre-hormone rather than a vitamin; it is transformed in the body into an active hormone. Although vitamins are very important for health, hormones are even more powerful. The active hormone is called calcitriol (or 1,25-dihydroxyvitamin D). Calcitriol has many important roles in the body.

Human DNA contains more than 2700 binding sites for activated vitamin D (or calcitriol) and over 200 genes are significantly influenced by activated vitamin D, with many of these 200 genes being related to autoimmune diseases, including MS.

Unlike all other vitamins, vitamin D is rare in standard human diets. The major source of vitamin D for most humans is sunlight, not food—even for those in less sunny countries. Hence, vitamin D deficiency and insufficiency are very common, with recent reports estimating that over one billion people are deficient or insufficient. This means that more than one in every eight people is affected at any time.

Vitamin D is essential for human health; however, a large proportion of the world's population has low levels of vitamin D

There is a dramatic difference between modern-day and pre-modern lifestyles. Nowadays we spend much more time indoors—most of us work indoors, socialise indoors, eat indoors, and so on. The switch to almost total indoor living means we have limited sun exposure and this restricts the biggest available source of vitamin D.

Let's first discuss the importance of vitamin D to general health and how to get enough of it. This will help prevent you from being one of the one billion people who don't have adequate vitamin D.

Why is vitamin D important?

Vitamin D is best known for its effects on bone health. Vitamin D increases calcium absorption from the food we eat, with calcium being an important component of bones. However, vitamin D has many other functions, including regulating inflammation and the immune system, and healthy brain function. In fact, there are vitamin D receptors in virtually all types of cells in the body and activated vitamin D can be made inside most tissues, including immune cells and the brain.

What are the symptoms of low vitamin D?

In children, prolonged vitamin D deficiency causes rickets, while in adults low vitamin D causes a condition called osteomalacia. Both of these conditions are the result of soft bones. Rickets was first described in Scotland during the industrial revolution where lack of sunlight, due to narrow streets and tall buildings preventing sun from reaching street level, pollution and the fact that many children worked indoors in factories all contributed to the increased incidence of low vitamin D levels and therefore childhood rickets. Rickets, while still relatively uncommon, is more prevalent today than it should be. Symptoms of low vitamin D are not always noticeable and can be quite general, such as fatigue, bone pain and weakness.

Who is at risk of low vitamin D?

As vitamin D is rare in standard human diets and sunshine is the largest contributor to the vitamin D status in most people, anyone who is unable to access or who avoids or limits sun exposure is at risk of low vitamin D levels. With this in mind, there are several major influences on vitamin D levels, including geography, season and sun-avoiding behaviours such as covering up and applying sunscreen.

However, there are some groups of people who may be at added risk of low vitamin D levels, including:

- dark-skinned individuals—the darker the skin, the more melanin pigment it contains and therefore the lower the efficiency of vitamin D production

- overweight or obese—vitamin D is a fat-soluble vitamin; as vitamin D is stored in body fat, the greater the body fat, the greater the need for vitamin D
- elderly—as we age, the capacity of our skin to produce vitamin D decreases
- less mobile individuals—may be less able to get out into the sun than those who are fully mobile
- people with liver or kidney disease—vitamin D, whether from sunlight, supplements or diet, is processed first in the liver and then in the kidneys or other tissues; for a person with severe liver or kidney disease, this can affect vitamin D processing
- people with conditions affecting fat malabsorption—conditions like inflammatory bowel disease and coeliac disease can result in lower levels of vitamin D.

Sunlight is not toxic; it is important for everyone to get regular sensible sun exposure, especially people with MS and other autoimmune diseases

Furthermore, some medications can decrease vitamin D absorption (e.g. anti-epileptic medications) or vitamin D processing (e.g. steroids).

Vitamin D and risk of MS

MS and location

Early studies in the middle of last century reported that MS rates were much higher in countries that were further away from the equator, such as the United Kingdom and Canada, than in countries closer to the equator, such as Columbia, Kenya and Malaysia. However, there are many differences between these countries aside from sun and vitamin D. Interest in sunlight and vitamin D with regards to MS began to grow when studies reported that even in the same country, MS rates were higher in areas of the country further from the equator. In New Zealand, for instance, there is a 300 per cent increase in MS rates in parts of the country further from the equator compared with parts closer to the equator.

In Australia, a much larger country, there is a six-fold difference between Queensland and Tasmania.

MS and season

Many features of MS may be associated with the time of year. For instance, people born in winter and whose birthplace is in low-sunshine areas develop MS symptoms years earlier than those born in seasons other than winter and in medium- and high-sunshine areas. MS relapses are also more common when there is less sunlight. This seasonal effect is particularly strong in countries where seasons are clearly different, with the highest MS rates occurring in spring (end of winter) and the lowest MS rates in autumn (end of summer). This is because vitamin D levels are high at the end of summer while vitamin D levels are low at the end of winter.

Vitamin D and MS progression

This isn't the place to review all the research showing how important it is to prevent low vitamin D levels for people with MS. Suffice to say it is a large evidence base, and the case is strong. The *Overcoming Multiple Sclerosis* book goes into that in some detail. In brief, the research shows that higher vitamin D levels are associated with a lower number of MS relapses. Even in those taking disease-modifying therapies, people with MS with lower vitamin D levels have higher relapse rates, and those with higher levels have slower MS progression, less active disease and less brain shrinkage. There is also evidence that there is a link between the genes involved in MS and the genes involved in vitamin D levels. This means that MS may actually reduce vitamin D levels, and people with MS may find it harder to raise their levels with supplements.

Some studies have shown that giving people with MS vitamin D supplements can reduce inflammation and promote an anti-inflammatory profile. Giving people with MS vitamin D supplements can also improve quality of life, especially mental health. Many small studies have found benefits for giving people with MS vitamin D supplements, including for relapse rates (particularly during winter when levels normally drop), a reduction in the number of brain lesions on MRI scans and slower progression of disability.

As we can see, vitamin D seems to be involved in the immune system and brain health and also directly involved in MS genesis and progression. In addition, many of the common symptoms of MS may also respond to vitamin D. These symptoms include depression or low mood and fatigue or low energy levels as well as cognitive function.

Low vitamin D levels predispose individuals to developing MS; for people with the disease, low levels are linked to disease progression and worsening of symptoms

Sun exposure and risk of MS

So there is a large and consistent body of research linking low sun exposure and subsequent low vitamin D levels to MS. However, the non–vitamin D benefits of sun exposure mean that low sun exposure itself is strongly related to MS risk.

Sun exposure modulates the immune system in many separate but positive ways, with direct benefits for risk of MS. We have long known that earlier life sun exposure (before adulthood) seems to have a lasting effect on general health but also the development and progression of MS. People who have higher sun exposure at an early age are much less likely to be diagnosed with MS. Even in the Arctic Circle, increased outdoor activities during summer in early life have been associated with about half the risk of MS. Again, winter sun exposure seems to be more important than summer sun exposure. This suggests that sunlight has benefits other than via vitamin D. Twin studies, important because identical twins have identical genes, have provided evidence that the protective effect of sun exposure in MS is independent of genetic susceptibility.

Many studies have shown that people with the lowest sun exposure, particularly in early life, have considerably greater odds of developing MS when compared with those with the highest sun exposure. Only part of this effect seems to be related to lower vitamin D levels. The sun seems to provide other direct benefits too.

Interestingly, research has revealed that for people diagnosed with a first-ever attack of MS (called, until there is evidence of further disease activity, 'clinically isolated syndrome' or CIS), higher sun exposure prior to this event was related to lower risk of progression to a full diagnosis of MS. And more sun exposure meant progressively less risk. Those who deliberately increased their sun exposure after the CIS diagnosis also had less risk of progression to a full MS diagnosis. One study examined MS rates compared to sun exposure in major cities across Australia and found that variation in MS rates was very closely related to sunshine levels—that is, higher sun meant less MS.

One very large study used two datasets comprising over 7000 people with MS and nearly 7000 control subjects without MS. Low sun exposure increased MS risk indirectly—that is, low sun exposure increased MS risk through low vitamin D levels. The research also found that low sun exposure increased MS risk directly—that is, less sun exposure increased MS risk through lack of immune modulation and other non-vitamin D factors. In fact, the researchers estimated that of the total beneficial effect of sun exposure, less than 30 per cent was due to vitamin D. It's clearly important to get sun exposure and not just take vitamin D.

Other studies have shown that sun exposure over the life course appears to reduce the risk of MS regardless of race and ethnicity, even for darker skinned people who raise their vitamin D levels less than pale-skinned people for any given amount of sun exposure.

Sun exposure and MS progression

There is evidence that MS is more severe in individuals in the same country if they live further from the equator and rates of death from MS are higher in countries further away from the equator. A growing number of studies have shown that people with MS enjoy many benefits of greater sun exposure, including less depression and fatigue, fewer relapses, and even lower death rates. Other research has suggested that sun exposure may be very important for those with progressive MS, not just those with the relapsing form.

Sun exposure has clear benefits for people with MS over and above its effect on raising vitamin D levels

Evidence for the actual part of sunlight that is responsible for these direct benefits for people with MS is still preliminary. However, as with vitamin D production, it appears that UV light may be the important part. One study showed that while vitamin D supplements did not prevent progression to diagnosed MS from CIS, treatment with UV light did. While still in the early stages, there is clearly supporting research to suggest that for people with MS there is a distinct benefit over and above taking vitamin D for sun and UV exposure.

So it is likely that vitamin D alone does not provide all the benefits of sunshine. In the same way that a vitamin C supplement is not the same as eating lots of fruit rich in vitamin C, sensible sun exposure seems to have multiple additional benefits compared with vitamin D alone. Here are some of the benefits of getting adequate sun exposure:

- UV rays from the sun have an immunomodulatory effect—meaning that the sun can actually modulate the immune system
- lack of vitamin D toxicity—it is not possible to get vitamin D toxicity from sun exposure; this is because the body stops making vitamin D after about 15–20 minutes of sun exposure
- modulation of the gut microbiome
- regulation of our circadian rhythm—in other words, our sleep–wake cycle, including through the hormone melatonin
- UV rays from the sun can increase the level of nitric oxide in the body; nitric oxide has many functions, one of which is to improve blood flow to the brain
- other—it is possible, even likely, that there are many undiscovered effects of sun exposure.

Is sunshine safe?

That excessive sunlight causes skin cancer is well accepted in medical science. Excessive sunshine also seems to contribute to eye problems and premature skin ageing. However, it is important to note that this does not mean sun should be avoided by everyone all of the time. Too much of any good thing can be bad—for example, water! Drinking too much water can be very harmful and even result in death but we don't advise people to never drink water.

Modern medical science actually concludes that complete avoidance of sun is not healthy and sensible sun exposure has multiple benefits for the therapy of many different types of common disease, including diabetes, thrombotic events such as stroke and a variety of cancers.

One Swedish study reported a twofold higher death rate among avoiders of sun exposure compared with the highest sun exposure group. In a follow-up study, the same group of researchers reported that the risk from avoidance of sun exposure was of a similar magnitude to the risk from smoking, and that compared with the highest sun exposure group, life expectancy of avoiders of sun exposure was reduced by 0.6–2.1 years! Interesting, isn't it? After all the public health advice we hear about avoiding sun, insufficient sun exposure seems to come with real health consequences. It has been estimated that as a result, there is a very large economic burden in the United States due to vitamin D insufficiency from inadequate sun exposure, poor diet and low take-up of supplements.

The evidence really stacks up. For people with MS, and for those at risk of MS, it's critical to receive adequate sun exposure and to maintain adequate vitamin D levels, and this frequently means supplementing with vitamin D. Now for the practical issues associated with achieving enough sun exposure, good vitamin D levels and the right supplementation of vitamin D. These things aren't actually difficult, but it's important to understand the detail so as not to risk too much sun or vitamin D from supplements on the one hand, or too little on the other.

How do I know if I have enough vitamin D?

The best and simplest way to know if you have enough vitamin D is to get a blood test. Most doctors and healthcare providers can arrange this type of test easily. The specific test is called 25-hydroxyvitamin D, which is often abbreviated to 25(OH)D, or just a vitamin D level.

Blood levels of vitamin D are measured in nanomoles per litre (nmol/L) in most parts of the world but in nanograms per millilitre (ng/mL) in the United States. To convert nanomoles per litre into nanograms per millilitre, simply divide by 2.5, and to convert nanograms per millilitre into nanomoles per litre, simply multiply by 2.5. Different health authorities recommend different 25(OH)D levels but a general rule is 75–225 nmol/L or 30–90 nanograms per millilitre.

The simplest way to tell if you are getting enough vitamin D is to have a blood test

It can take several months for your vitamin D level to stabilise after commencing a vitamin D supplement. Therefore, it is wise to supplement daily on a consistent basis before getting your vitamin D level checked. The vitamin D blood level after 3–4 months of supplementation will tell you if your supplement dose is too low, too high or just right.

How do we get vitamin D?

There are three broad sources of vitamin D: sun, supplements and diet, in that order of importance.

Sun

When we look at populations, vitamin D levels are highest at the end of summer and lowest at the end of winter. So countries in the northern hemisphere—for example, Ireland, the United Kingdom and the United States—tend to have the highest vitamin D levels in September and the lowest levels in March. It is important to point out that the specific component of sunshine responsible for vitamin D production is called ultraviolet B radiation, or simply UVB.

It is possible to get UVB from some types of lamps and sun beds but these are complicated and controversial. For example, the World Health Organization lists artificial sun beds as a class-one carcinogen—carcinogen meaning cancer-causing and class one meaning highest levels of evidence. Therefore, for the rest of this chapter I will refer to UVB simply as sun.

Sun exposure is such a powerful influence in vitamin D production that controlled studies have shown a single 20-minute exposure to sunlight in a bathing suit can produce up to 20,000 international units (IU) of vitamin D. In terms of food, this is the equivalent of consuming 2.5 kilograms (5 lbs 8 oz) of salmon, 500 large eggs or 100 glasses of fortified milk!

However, it is important to note that the human body is very smart, so although we can gain lots of vitamin D from sun exposure, humans cannot receive too much from sun alone. This is because the body shuts off production of vitamin D when we have enough.

Darker skin has the same capacity but less efficiency to produce vitamin D. What this means is that it is certainly possible for someone with darker skin to produce vitamin D but it takes longer. Also, darker skin is less susceptible to sun damage and therefore a person with darker skin can safely expose themselves to sun for longer than a person with lighter skin.

This is all fine when a person lives in a sunny location and can get out in the sun regularly. But it is problematic when a person does not live in a sunny location or cannot access the sun regularly. On the flipside, someone with very pale skin may be able to produce vitamin D very efficiently but may avoid sun because of a tendency to burn quickly.

So lighter skin means more efficient vitamin D production from sun but more chance of skin damage, while darker skin means less-efficient vitamin D production from sun but less chance of skin damage. Regardless of skin type, everybody should consider a vitamin D supplement when sun exposure is not possible, as is the case in many parts of the world in winter.

Sun exposure is the best source of vitamin D

The major factors affecting vitamin D production from sunlight are as follows:

- Duration of exposure—humans produce more vitamin D from longer exposure, up to about 20 minutes per body area; think of 10–15 minutes with the front of your body facing the sun and 10–15 minutes with your back facing the sun.
- Time of day—for humans to be able to produce vitamin D, the sun needs to be relatively strong so think of 10–15 minutes near the middle of the day as opposed to very early in the morning or late in the day when the sun will be weaker.
- Time of year—in most parts of the world, to get the same amount of vitamin D in winter, you will need to get more sun exposure than in summer; in some places further from the equator, you won't get any vitamin D at all in winter.
- Cloud cover—clouds can partially block UV rays from reaching the earth's surface.
- Latitude—in other words, distance from the equator; you may only need to stay out in the sun at midday for a few minutes in Singapore regardless of time of year compared with, say, Boston where you need to stay out much longer; and won't get any vitamin D no matter how long you stay out in winter.
- Amount of skin exposed—wearing a tracksuit with only hands and face exposed will produce only a fraction of what is produced if wearing a swimsuit.
- Sunscreen—can block over 90 per cent of vitamin D production; put sunscreen on after about 15 minutes of sun exposure if staying out for longer periods.
- Age of the person—as we age, we produce less vitamin D from sunshine.
- Frequency—how often you get out in sunlight.

Kerley's rule for sun exposure

I summarise my own rules for sun exposure as follows:

1. Short shadow.
2. More skin, less time.
3. Never burn.

Short shadow

A good rule of thumb is that when your shadow is shorter than your body, you are capable of making adequate amounts of vitamin D. However, when your shadow is longer than your body, you are not capable of making sufficient vitamin D. This is because when the sun is high in the sky and almost straight overhead, the UV rays can reach the earth's surface. But when the sun is low in the sky and your shadow is long, most UV rays do not reach the earth's surface. So no matter where in the world you are, what time of year it is or what time of day it is, check how long your shadow is for an easy way to assess whether the sun is strong enough for vitamin D production.

More skin, less time

Try to expose more skin for a shorter period of time rather than a little skin for a long time. This means going out in the sun in shorts and a vest or a swimming suit for 10–60 minutes (less in summer, more in winter) rather than going out in trousers and a shirt with only face and hands exposed for hours at a time. Remember that if you have darker skin you will need longer in the sun to make vitamin D. A total of 10–20 minutes of sun exposure might be enough for most people with lighter skin but 45–60 minutes might be required for somebody with darker skin. Exposing more skin for less time means you can maximise vitamin D production while minimising damage from excessive sun. This is something that is often not mentioned in standard public health messages.

Never burn

There can be no doubt that too much sun can be harmful. However, sensible sun exposure has many benefits for overall health and specifically with regards to MS. Further, throughout history, humans have always been exposed to the sun. The most harmful aspect of sun exposure is sunburn. We should always try to avoid getting burned from excessive sun exposure. Some people may avoid sun because there is a risk. It is important to remember that almost everything has a risk—as I have mentioned, even too much water can cause death! But people still drink water because it is vital for life. Similarly, there is no need to avoid sun exposure altogether, just be sensible and always avoid burning. Like water, the sun is also vital for health.

Vitamin D supplements

Look for a vitamin D–only supplement

As I've said, a major role for vitamin D is in promoting bone health and increasing calcium absorption. However, some vitamin D supplements also contain calcium. It is not advisable to supplement vitamin D and calcium at the same time. This may well cause a serious side effect: high blood-calcium levels or hypercalcaemia. Although hypercalcaemia can be treated if caught early, it can progress and be very severe. There is now, in fact, some evidence that taking calcium supplements in general can be harmful to health, potentially causing an increased risk of diseases associated with blood clotting such as heart disease and stroke.

Vitamin D2 vs D3

There are two main types of vitamin D: vitamin D2, also called ergocalciferol; and vitamin D3, also called cholecalciferol. Vitamin D2 is completely absent from humans who do not supplement with vitamin D2. Vitamin D3 is the type of vitamin D that we produce in our skin from sunlight exposure. Vitamin D3 is also the type of vitamin D found in fatty fish such as salmon, mackerel and sardines.

Although vitamin D2 can increase vitamin D levels, there is a wealth of scientific evidence that vitamin D3 is more effective than vitamin D2 with respect to its benefits for a variety of health conditions, and it is likely that MS falls into the same category. Most supplements contain vitamin D3 or cholecalciferol but make sure you check the label to be sure.

To ensure year-round adequate vitamin D levels, vitamin D3 supplements are needed in winter in many parts of the world

What determines our response to vitamin D sources?

The response of every individual to vitamin D from the sun, supplements, diet or a combination of all three is variable. The major factors influencing our blood levels of vitamin D are frequency of sun exposure or vitamin D supplementation, dose, body size (larger individuals require more vitamin D; this is true for individuals who are overweight, very tall or very muscular) and individual variation. A blood test is the best way to see whether you are getting enough.

Is vitamin D safe?

Yes, vitamin D is very safe. But like most healthy and beneficial substances, too much can cause harm. However, this is *not* a reason to avoid vitamin D supplements or be afraid. As I have said, one cannot get too much vitamin D from the sun. But it is possible to overdose on supplements. For people getting a lot of sun exposure, the dose of supplements needs to be lower to achieve the same blood level. However, it has been determined that the safe tolerable upper limit of dosing of vitamin D3 for humans is 10,000 IU per day, regardless of sun exposure. In practice, however, for people who get a lot of sun, taking this much will result in a blood level that is above the upper limit of 225 nmol/L. It can get as high as 350 nmol/L. While there have been no reported cases of toxicity from people taking this level of supplementation, it is wise to reduce the dose when getting a lot of sun. The OMS Program recommends taking up to 10,000 IU a day in winter in places where there isn't much sun and up to 5,000 IU a day in summer.

Signs and symptoms of vitamin D toxicity

The first sign of vitamin D toxicity is hypercalciuria (too much calcium in the urine), followed by hypercalcaemia (too much calcium in the blood).

The immediate symptoms of vitamin D overdose are:

• abdominal cramps, nausea, vomiting and lack of appetite, which can all lead to weight loss

- excess urination with dehydration and thirst
- conjunctivitis (symptom of dehydration)
- bowel issues, including constipation or diarrhoea
- weakness
- tingling mouth sensations
- confusion
- abnormal heartbeat (arrhythmia)
- kidney issues, including kidney stones, hardening of the blood vessels in the kidneys (calcification) and even kidney failure.

Vitamin D supplementation is very safe in doses of up to 10,000 IU a day; less is required for people who get plenty of sun

None of these is likely to occur if sticking with the recommendations here and in the *Overcoming Multiple Sclerosis* book.

Diet

The reason that diet is listed last is that it is the least important source of vitamin D. It is extremely difficult to get all of our vitamin D needs from natural foods alone. I specify 'natural' because many foods can be fortified with vitamin D, such as soy milk or breakfast cereals. However, overall, healthy foods such as vegetables and fruit contain literally zero vitamin D. In fact, the only major natural source of vitamin D is oily fish such as salmon, sardines and mackerel. White fish such as cod and whiting contain considerably less vitamin D than oily varieties. Some mushrooms do contain vitamin D but these need to have been exposed to sunshine. Even then mushrooms will contain vitamin D2, while vitamin D3 is preferred for humans. A large serving of vitamin D-enriched mushrooms can contain only around 350 IU, and of course they can be expensive.

How to implement this knowledge?

There is now a large and coherent body of research reporting that vitamin D and sun exposure have a crucial role in MS, both in terms of the risk of developing the disease and in terms of its progression and effects. It seems that both are important and people with MS should ideally aim for both. Strive for regular and sensible sun exposure when possible and practical. Of course, this may not be easy, depending on your location. If it is difficult for you to get sensible and regular sun exposure, make sure your vitamin D intake and levels are regularly monitored. It's one of the easiest and simplest steps in the OMS Program, but one that is commonly forgotten.

Ground covered

Modern indoor lifestyles make it hard for most people to get adequate sun exposure. This leads to low vitamin D levels for many people, with serious health consequences, including an increased risk of developing MS. For those with MS, it can lead to worsening of symptoms and progression of the disease.

Getting adequate sun exposure is very safe in moderation, and has many benefits for people with MS. In most parts of the world, sun exposure in winter is insufficient to improve health; this will necessitate supplementing with vitamin D.

Vitamin D supplements are safe up to an upper limit of 10,000 IU a day. The best way of telling if you are taking enough is to get a blood test.

My Story: Emma Lister

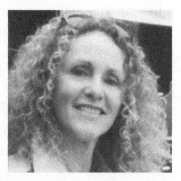

My MS story began in 2004, unknowingly, with vision loss and stabbing eye pain. Pain from neck and back disc injuries over a period of ten years masked the worsening back pain, spasms and weakness that in hindsight were presumably related to underlying MS. I underwent MRI scans, osteopathic and chiropractic treatments and intense physiotherapy rehabilitation to regain use of my gluteal muscles and legs, taking anti-inflammatories and other pain relief to help dampen my overwhelming symptoms.

Early in 2016 my torso began to feel like it was being crushed: I was experiencing prickling pain, and started to lose power in my legs. Later that year I received the life-changing diagnosis of relapsing remitting MS after previous symptoms had been labelled optic neuritis and transverse myelitis. Although devastating, there was relief in finally getting an answer after years of struggling. But equally I was determined to find a way to overcome this.

At the end of that year, my new yoga teacher offered advice that would change my life. 'Google Professor George Jelinek and you won't look back,' she said. That's exactly what I did. After 72 hours of reading *Overcoming Multiple Sclerosis* and *Recovering from Multiple Sclerosis*, with kitchen cupboards cleared, I began the OMS Program. The science made total sense! Highly motivated, desperate to regain my life, I set off on my journey with an 'all or nothing approach'. I thought that if all these people could recover, so could I.

On diagnosis my vitamin D levels had been a little low at 138 nmol/L, so I immediately started taking two sprays per day of 3000 IU oral vitamin D and also increasing sun exposure to 20 minutes per day without sunscreen. I felt like I was finally in the driver's seat, organising blood tests annually at the end of February. My levels increased to 166 nmol/L in 2017, then to 175 nmol/L in 2018—a level that I have maintained to the current day. I now feel confident that I am able to maintain and control my vitamin D levels. Being able to ski again also offered an excellent additional source of vitamin D in the darker winter months.

Within six weeks of starting the Program, I remarkably overcame approximately twenty symptoms. My Lhermitte's disappeared (this is an uncomfortable sensation that can travel from your neck down your spine), normal bladder and bowel function returned, there was huge visual improvement, my eye and facial twitching ceased, and I enjoyed improvement in many other symptoms, to the point where I was able to walk and even jog upstairs without pain. I achieved this through daily meditation and using yoga breathing/visualisation, eradicating the most painful problem first, working through the symptoms like peeling back an onion.

Upon returning to riding horses, my passion, I started to feel those wonderful endorphin and oxytocin rushes and my pain and stress began to dissipate.

Eventually I found a neurologist who understood my journey on the OMS Program and supported me on the road I had embarked upon. I felt that I was confidently standing my ground, instead of veering off down some unhelpful paths. I kept on track daily, using my OMS diary to write plans and record achievements.

The OMS charity and community have empowered me with abundant support, encouragement and hope. The OMS Ammerdown retreat in 2018 was undoubtedly an incredible, life-changing experience. Cocooned within an overwhelming sense of warmth, I felt like I truly belonged in the OMS community. Feeling so well and relapse-free, I wanted to give something back. So I trained and walked the 28-kilometre Thames Path Challenge later in 2018 with the wonderful OMS team to raise funds for the charity to show my appreciation.

Without the OMS Program, I have no doubt I would not be as healthy as I am today. Amazingly, in June 2020 I was 'signed off' by my neurologist because I am so well. I didn't realise that such a thing could happen.

The OMS Program has given me my life back, for which I am eternally grateful. Thank you.

5

Exercise

Dr Stuart White

> No matter your ability, making any form of exercise
> as much of a habit as eating and breathing will be
> something that your future self will look back and
> smile upon.
>
> *Alexander Tsirigotis, London, UK*

Often, the first shock finding after a diagnosis of MS is that the
illness is incurable. This is usually followed by a realisation that
your ability to walk might get worse over time. It is normal to
feel afraid about how the disease will affect you physically: How
will I get around? How will other people judge me walking differently? Will I fall over more? How will my life be restricted? Will
I end up in a wheelchair? Will I be able to do things for myself?
Will I end up relying on other people?

You can also find yourself wondering how you are going to
carry on doing the sports that you enjoy. How can I enjoy running
if walking is affected? How can I enjoy cycling if balance is
affected? How can I enjoy the gym, or gardening, if mobility
is affected?

These concerns are very understandable, but a diagnosis of
MS does not mean that you are automatically going to get worse
physically and end up in a wheelchair. Indeed, by following the
OMS Program you can help yourself avoid this outcome. People
with MS very commonly report that the Program has given them

a much better understanding of the importance of looking after themselves physically and making exercise a vital part of their new lifestyle.

Many studies over several years have shown that exercise improves people's physical and mental health, and quality of life. This applies to people with MS too. The HOLISM study is one of a large and growing number of research studies that has looked specifically at exercise in people with MS. These studies have found a number of key associations between better physical *and* mental health and regular exercise, including better general fitness, increased muscle strength, less disability, better bowel and bladder function, less fatigue, better mood and concentration, fewer other illnesses and improved quality of life. Also, it is reassuring that many of these studies have shown that exercise has very few downsides and does not seem to make people's MS worse. On the contrary, regular exercise improves the course of MS: to paraphrase the old saying, 'If exercise were a pill, everyone would be taking it'.

Regular exercise reduces the risk of developing other common diseases such as heart disease, obesity, diabetes, dementia, cancer and autoimmune diseases, which can worsen MS

In this chapter we will look at why, how and how much people with MS should exercise, as well as how to overcome the physical and mental barriers that people with MS might have about doing regular exercise (such as overheating, using physical aids and worrying about injury).

Why should I exercise?

On some level everyone understands that exercise is good for health and wellbeing. You may have read or heard about the latest research describing its benefits in newspapers or on television. You might be training to take part in competitive sport. You may feel great after walking the dog, running around in the park with your children or cycling to work.

There is now a large amount of scientific research that consistently shows that exercise maintains wellness and prevents illness. But increasingly, scientists are realising that regular exercise prevents physical illnesses from getting worse. Also, scientists have started to rediscover that regular physical exercise is an essential part of mental and psychological wellbeing, and improves overall quality of life ('*mens sana in corpore sano*'— 'a healthy mind in a healthy body').

Regular exercise improves the physical and mental health, and quality of life, of people with MS

Importantly for diseases like MS, exercise has specific, helpful effects on the nervous system. Exercise:

- increases some chemicals, such as brain-derived neurotrophic factor (BDNF) and nerve-growth factor (NGF), which protect the brain against damage and promote the growth of new nerve cells
- decreases other chemicals, such as interleukin-17 and gamma-interferon, reducing inflammation by dampening the body's immune cells. It appears to create an environment in the brain that helps damaged nerve cells to remyelinate
- improves the ability of the brain to form new nerve pathways, which allow it to constantly adapt itself and compensate for the damage caused by MS (this is called 'neuroplasticity'); the more complex the exercise, the greater the adaptation
- lessens brain inflammation, thereby reducing fatigue, depression and 'brain fog'
- improves sleep and metabolism, helping you to rest and recover
- reduces stress
- helps regulate weight and appetite.

Finally, many people with MS find that exercise has a spiritual benefit. There is something incredibly reassuring about taking control of MS, doing things both to manage symptoms and to stop the condition from getting worse. MS is a condition that most often affects how much and how well you can move your body. So taking part in regular exercise reminds you of how much you *can* do physically, rather than what you *can't* do, and helps you find ways of overcoming symptoms that affect mind and body. People with MS find this particularly important as they grow older: it can be difficult to determine whether any physical symptoms are caused by age or MS, or both, but regular exercise helps to overcome symptoms caused by both.

What confuses many people is just *why* exercise works. After all, exercise causes inflammation, and we think of inflammation as generally being bad for people, particularly people with MS.

Exercise places stress on the body. Some chemicals released into the bloodstream during exercise act as signals for the body to repair itself and prepare itself for exercise in the future. Some of these chemicals cause 'acute' inflammation, lasting a few days. In the 'repair' days shortly after exercise, this will be felt as stiffness or soreness. In the 'prepare' days after that, the body adapts to deal with further exercise. It does this, for example, by increasing the ability of the heart to pump blood, of the lungs to breathe in oxygen, of the immune system to function and how hard and long the muscles are able to work for. This adaptation is known as 'conditioning'.

Exercise causes acute inflammation over days, which produces healthy adaptations in the body; lack of exercise contributes to chronic inflammation over years, which leads to illness

The opposite, known as 'deconditioning', can occur when you stop exercising or do not exercise at all. Together with poor diet and stress, lack of exercise worsens body function, and makes you more likely to get common diseases as you get older, such as heart disease, obesity, diabetes, dementia, cancer and autoimmune diseases. These illnesses involve 'chronic' inflammation lasting years to decades. Furthermore, developing these illnesses can worsen MS.

What exercise is best?

When exercising, the body combines glucose (that is eaten) with oxygen (that is breathed in) to produce energy (so muscles work), water (which is peed out) and carbon dioxide (which is breathed out). This is called 'aerobic' ('with air') respiration, and is mainly what powers muscles for longer-lasting, endurance exercises (such as walking, running and cycling). Aerobic exercise is good for heart, lung and blood vessel function.

As you exercise harder and harder, there comes a point when you can't make enough energy aerobically, and so the body makes extra energy without oxygen (but less efficiently). This is called 'anaerobic' ('without air') respiration, and is what helps power muscles during short, sharp strength exercises (such as weightlifting, and sprinting during aerobic exercise). Anaerobic exercise is good for bone and muscle strength.

Below the 'anaerobic threshold' you produce energy aerobically. Above the anaerobic threshold, you produce energy aerobically and anaerobically. You know roughly when you have reached the anaerobic threshold during exercise because you feel your muscles start to burn. To get fitter, you need to do mostly aerobic but also some anaerobic exercise. Some types of exercise are naturally aerobic and anaerobic at the same time, such as swimming, boxing and gardening.

Generally, every week *any* adult should aim for three aerobic exercise days, two anaerobic exercise days and two rest days. Aerobic sessions should last 1–2 hours, anaerobic sessions about one hour. If you don't exercise much (or at all), this can seem like a lot but is actually quite easy to incorporate into a busy life. We'll discuss how you might do this below.

People with MS need to do some stamina exercise, some strength exercise, some balance exercise and some stretching, each week

More specifically, there are types of exercise that people with MS should also do to offset some of the effects of MS. In particular, stretching exercises can help overcome spasticity and muscle tightness, and balance exercises help with walking and avoiding falls. Stretching and balance exercises include yoga and Pilates.

If they occur, physical symptoms in people with MS are usually more common in the lower half of the body than the upper half. Everyone with MS has slightly different symptoms. It's important to do regular exercise for its many physical and mental benefits; but it is also important to do exercises that compensate for getting older, or according to how your MS symptoms are changing. How are you going to carry on moving your body as the years go by? What exercises do you need to do now and in the future for 'functional fitness'? For example, what do you need to physically be able to do to: carry on working (Do you have to commute? How much do you have to carry and for how long?); look after children (Can you pick them up? Can you play with them?); look after yourself (How will you get around? How will you shop?)? You can follow special exercise plans for these 'activities of daily living', which can also be important when setting goals for making exercise more enjoyable.

How much exercise is appropriate?

Exercise improves health and wellbeing in people with MS, but only up to a point. With exercise, there is a sweet spot between 'just enough' (where you get all the benefits) and 'too much' (where you get injured or lose interest). Figure 5.1 shows these effects.

Too much exercise can be as harmful as too little exercise. Remember that exercise causes stress to the body, and it's the body's adaptation to this stress that delivers the health benefits. Adaptation actually takes place when resting between episodes of exercise—if you don't rest for long enough, you don't adapt to exercise, and you won't get as many health benefits (as well as making injury more likely).

Of course, the shape of this curve is different for everyone. Most people have a similarly shaped fitness curve, but vary where they start from or how much exercise they need to benefit from it. A small number of people are 'super-responders' with narrow curves, who are able to get very fit with little exercise. Similarly, a small number of people are 'non-responders' with flat curves, who don't get much fitter (or get sicker) no matter how much exercise they do. Most of us are somewhere in between these extremes, and so we need to work to get fit, and work hard to get very fit.

Like much of the OMS Program, what is important here is that *you yourself* need to experiment to find what works best for you, in this case reaching that sweet spot where enough exercise gives you the most benefit.

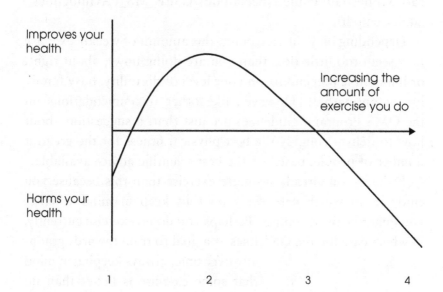

Figure 5.1: Exercise, but don't overexercise. This graph holds roughly true for both a single exercise session and for exercise overall as part of an OMS lifestyle. Starting at '1', the graph shows that not exercising at all can be harmful to overall health. As you start exercising, even small amounts of exercise improve health, towards a 'sweet spot' at point 2, where the exercise effort you are putting in has the most benefit for health. However, as you do more exercise, you start to see diminishing returns (point 3). If you push your body even further towards point 4, you start to harm yourself with exercise by not recovering between physical efforts, and/or injuring yourself.

Even small amounts of exercise will improve health compared with not exercising at all

Several sets of up-to-date guidelines recommend what types of exercise people with MS should do every week, and for how long. These are based on studies of how much exercise people with MS seem to need to remain physically fit. For adults aged 18–64 with MS of mild/moderate severity, for example, the Canadian Society of Exercise Physiology recommends 30 minutes of moderately intense aerobic activity twice a week and two sets of 10–15 repetitions of strength training exercises for major muscle groups twice a week (http://csep.ca/CMFiles/Guidelines/specialpops/CSEP_MS_PAGuidelines_adults_en.pdf).

Depending on your viewpoint, this amount of weekly exercise may seem too little (less than you are doing now), about right, or impossible (depending on your level of disability, busy family life or antipathy!). However, like other recommendations on the OMS Program, guidelines are just that: a suggestion about how to deliver roughly the best physical fitness for the greatest number of people, based on the best scientific advice available.

Perhaps you already do more exercise than this because you enjoy it, in which case carry on (but keep in mind whether you might be overtraining). Perhaps you do no exercise currently, in which case use the guidelines as a goal to train towards gradually over time, always keeping in mind that some exercise is better than no exercise at all. Perhaps you feel that the amount of exercise you do is about right, in which case reassess whether this is the case: Could you try some new exercise routines? Could you alter the ratio of strength and endurance training you do, to reach a new goal? Could you learn a new exercise skill?

You need to find the balance between exercising enough to get the most health benefit, but not too much so that your health suffers

Overcoming barriers to regular exercise

A wealth of research evidence shows the benefits of exercise for people in general and for people with MS in particular. Perhaps rather than ask ourselves, 'Why exercise?', we should really be asking ourselves, 'Exercise— why not, indeed?!' Exercise should be a normal part of our lifestyle, rather than something that needs to be constantly added into our routine.

Worryingly, only an estimated 20 per cent of people with MS exercise regularly at all, compared with 40 per cent of the general population. Not exercising, however, leads to a spiral of downward decline. Inactivity leads to further disability and a higher chance of developing other illnesses (these were mentioned before: heart disease, obesity, diabetes, dementia, cancer and autoimmune diseases), which worsen disability and illness and make it harder to exercise, and so on.

Most people with MS should aim for about 5–8 hours of moderate (and occasionally vigorous) activity every week to get the maximum physical, mental and quality-of-life benefits from exercise

Determining why people with MS don't exercise can be difficult. A wide range of factors can prevent us from becoming involved in physical activity, or continuing to exercise regularly once we've started. A number of these might apply at the same time, and some are easier to identify than others. Most commonly, these barriers are mental: we listen to our brain excusing us from exercise, rather than listening to our body demanding we move and get active.

Hopefully by now, though, it will be clear that the OMS Program encourages a 'growth mindset'. It accepts that MS throws up all sorts of barriers to a normal life, but crucially, it also provides a positive way of thinking about how to overcome those barriers.

The stories we tell ourselves about why we can't exercise are always worth looking at again. Do they *really* hold true? Or could we make a few small changes that let us tell a better story about ourselves (and then make a few more changes, and then a few more)?

Take the word 'exercise' itself, for example. Words can be powerful, and carry huge meaning. Ask yourself, for example, does the word 'exercise' carry positive connotations of 'fun, feeling good, anticipation, necessity' for you, or does it carry negative ideas of 'pain, drudgery, shame and indifference'? Unsurprisingly, if you feel positive about it, you're more likely to exercise than if you feel negative. So don't call it 'exercise': try calling it 'movement' instead, or call it what it is ('walking', 'running', 'cycling', 'gym session'). Call it whatever word makes you happier to do it ('playtime'!).

More often than not, we learn to link words with meaning when we are young. You may have learned to link 'exercise' with 'pain', for example, on school cross-country runs, or with 'shame' from always being the last to get picked for school teams. People with MS who leave the school system with positive experiences tend to carry on with sport and exercise, or find it easy to restart these after their diagnosis. People with MS who leave with negative experiences tend not to exercise and find it hard to start exercising.

However much we think we can't change, though, we do change. A diagnosis of MS is a case in point: yesterday, you were 'you', today you're 'you with MS'. Change can force itself on you, but you can also force yourself to change. You have been diagnosed with MS, exercise will help you, and therefore you need to build exercise into your life.

Try telling a different story about yourself and exercise. For example, instead of thinking, 'I hate exercise, no matter how good it is for me', try telling yourself, 'I enjoy playing soccer with my kids in the park and it makes me fit'. Or what about reframing 'I'm afraid of falling over in the gym' as 'I like going to Pilates classes with my friend, and my balance has become a lot better'?

Listed on the following pages are some common barriers that stop people with MS from taking regular exercise, and how you might consider overcoming them. If you recognise them, think about how you could reframe them in a more positive way.

'I don't like exercise'

So what type of physical activity do you enjoy? Human beings didn't evolve to do triathlons or lift dumbbells, but to move around and engage with their surroundings. Think about physical activities you enjoy (dog walking). Start doing them (once a day). Start doing them more regularly (twice a day). Think about how to do them more strenuously (further, faster), add some complexity (play fetch!), and—hey, presto!—you're exercising.

'I haven't got the time to exercise'

I'm busy with work. I'm busy with the kids. I'm busy looking after my parents. I've got a busy social life. Busy, busy, busy! When you tell yourself that you're too busy to fit exercise into your lifestyle, you're really telling yourself that you think other things are more important, more worthy of your limited time, than looking after yourself. An MS diagnosis changes that story. Remember: you have been diagnosed with MS, exercise will help you, and therefore you need to build exercise into your life. Reprioritise!

Again, make small changes. Then add in some more small changes. And then some more, involving more effort and more complexity. Keep asking yourself: 'How can I mix exercise into this?' Too busy looking after kids? Younger kids love moving: move with them. So do older kids (and husbands/wives), especially when you explain to them why you need to get active and how you need their help to do so. It can be difficult to change other people, but *you can change* what you do. Commuting? Try building in longer and longer walks to your job and at lunchtime. Housework? Stretch more, lift more. Still short of time? Try compound exercises like swimming or gardening that involve aerobic and anaerobic exercise, and stretching. Make up your own gym routine with compound exercises (rowing, elliptical trainer, deadlift, push-up, pull-up) or ask a qualified fitness trainer for their advice.

'I can't afford to go to the gym'

Gyms can be expensive, certainly. Try talking to the gym management: they may offer reduced rates for different people at different times, and may accept a doctor's prescription (your private health insurance may cover gym membership). Of course, you don't have to go to the gym to get fit: get outside, move your body and have fun doing it.

'I'm too embarrassed', 'I'm too tired', 'I'm too sad', 'I get too hot'

These are really common problems for people with MS, and can be very difficult to admit to yourself and others. Not knowing how to exercise, and being older, overweight or visibly disabled can definitely make it more difficult to start an exercise plan, or keep it going once started. Again, though, only you can change yourself: one of the things that MS teaches us is to worry less about what other people (probably) are(n't) thinking of us when we're doing what we can to stay well.

Likewise, having a physical disability, tiredness or depression can make exercise more challenging, especially if you feel worse when you get hot (see pages 101–3). But ask yourself: not doing exercise—has it worked for you so far? Are you less stiff, tired and down? Is your balance any better? Or could you try changing things, doing more exercise and seeing how your mental and physical health, and quality of life improve? Be brave, be strong and keep turning up.

'I might get injured'

Both falls themselves and the fear of falling over are common for people with MS. Approximately 60 per cent of us have fallen over within the past six months, and 30 per cent of these have fallen more than once and been injured. It takes time to recover from a broken bone, which can reduce physical fitness further, and prevent exercise. It's unlikely that you will fall over when you are exercising. Instead, it is far more likely that regular exercise will considerably reduce your risk of falling as well as the risk of injuring yourself if you do fall.

A trained physical therapist can help design a safe exercise program that will allow you to target particular problems with mobility and avoid injury.

You can learn specific exercises to improve balance, leg strength, walking speed, body awareness, correct use of walking aids and bone strength. Indeed, falls and fracture prevention are such a problem worldwide that there are even specific exercises that can teach you how to fall better and avoid injury, based on martial arts moves.

'I might make my MS worse'

In the past, people with MS were told to avoid exercise in case it made their MS (symptoms) worse. There is no scientific evidence for this: exercise is not harmful for people with MS and does not cause MS relapses. In fact, the opposite appears to be true. Regular exercise seems to slow MS progression, in addition to all the other benefits mentioned previously (improved physical and mental fitness, better general health and improved quality of life).

How to start exercising regularly

So you need to build regular exercise into your new OMS lifestyle if you want to slow down the disease, and overcome its symptoms. Some will have been regular exercisers before diagnosis, and others may have already started exercising after diagnosis. However, you might want to exercise more effectively, or with more focus on certain exercises to improve symptoms.

Many, however, may find exercise the most difficult step of the OMS Program to tackle. That's completely fine: we all find one of the steps more difficult than the others. But tackle it *you must*. How do you change into becoming someone who exercises regularly? Here are the five Cs that people with MS commonly find helpful in doing this:

1. **Commit.** Remember, only you can change, and you can only change if you want to. If you commit yourself to doing more exercise, you will find a way. Every journey starts with a single step. Even small amounts of exercise are better than

none, and it is easier to build in more exercise to your life once you've already started.

2. **Check.** Check with your doctor, check with your family, check what facilities are available and check whether anyone can guide the exercise (e.g. qualified personal trainers or specialist MS physical therapists). View any problems that come up in these checks as barriers to overcome rather than barriers that stop you from exercising.

3. **Change** . . . slowly, but often. Occasionally, people can completely change their lifestyles overnight, and sometimes make those changes stick. Most of us have better success if we change our lifestyles slowly, however. We are aiming to form a regular exercise habit in our lives, and positive habits often take several months to harden. We know why we want to exercise, we know what the rewards will be and we've committed to change—so change! Pick something physical that you enjoy doing and that you can achieve. Call it exercise. Just start. Do it again. Do it harder, do it more often. Add difficulty. Learn a new skill. Feel the benefit. Add in some other 'exercises' that you enjoy. Over time, you've built exercise into your life . . .

4. **Be Consistent.** Remember that exercise is a lifestyle choice within the OMS Program—that is, it is something that you need to do regularly if you want to feel all of its benefits. It can be quite easy to fall out of the habit of exercise, and excuse ourselves from doing it ('it's too cold/wet out', 'I'm on holiday', 'my friends stopped coming with me').

Some of the best ways to reinforce the exercise habit involve socialising and goal-setting. Many people find that exercising with other people increases their enjoyment of it and their commitment to doing it regularly. Exercise classes, sports clubs, gyms, park runs, family walks—all of these, and others, provide the social support and reassurance that can help increase the fun of the activity. Exercise is play—play hard!

Goal-setting is a really great way of directing your efforts when you exercise. Ask yourself *regularly*: 'What do I want to achieve by exercising?' and 'How do I get there?' Remember that exercise goals may change with age and function—for example, from play when you're young, to competitive sport, leisure, daily activity and falls prevention as you get older, to independent mobility and living when you retire from work.

5. **Care.** Remember to reward yourself for meeting exercise goals, but also remember not to beat yourself up if you don't. For some people, beneficial habits like regular exercise can be harder to form than harmful habits, and take longer. Even with the best intentions, forming a regular exercise habit can be difficult at the first attempt, but you haven't failed if you've tried. Do you need to overcome different barriers? Do you need to make other changes? Can you ask other people to help you?

    Finally, take care not to overdo it. Aim for that sweet spot, and avoid diminishing returns and harm (see Figure 5.1): you can't exercise if you're injured. Be kind to yourself.

> *The 5 'Cs' approach can help you build regular exercise into your life: commit, check, change (slowly, but often), be consistent (set goals), care (be kind to yourself)*

Temperature management

About 60–80 per cent of us find that our MS symptoms get worse when we get hot. This is known as Uhthoff's phenomenon. We might notice that walking becomes more difficult when we get a fever, for example, or that we get tired more easily on hotter days. We might also notice that cooling ourselves down again brings our symptoms back to normal, and in some people, improves them.

The more you move and the harder you exercise, the more heat your body produces, and this can limit the amount of exercise you are able to do in one go. This is because electrical impulses move more slowly along damaged nerves as your body temperature increases, often affecting the ability to walk, balance and/or

Getting hot can make exercise more difficult

concentrate. The problem is made worse if you exercise hard indoors or in warmer climates.

Many of us find the effects of body heat on our ability to exercise very frustrating, and many people with MS avoid hot weather and exercise altogether. However, as we have seen above, exercising regularly produces important health benefits for people with MS. Dealing with MS into the future, therefore, means learning how to manage body temperature to avoid overheating, but also learning how to cool down safely.

A number of options exist, and it's worth experimenting to find which one works best for you. These include:

- Type of exercise—aerobic exercise (like running) tends to cause greater and longer increases in body temperature than shorter bouts of anaerobic exercise (like weightlifting), with fewer chances to cool down. Both strength and endurance exercise are important, but you may have to manage body temperature differently depending on the type of exercise.
- Where you exercise—try exercising outdoors on cool-weather days, and indoors on warm-weather days.
- When you exercise—mornings are generally cooler. Body temperature rises naturally in the evenings, and during the second half of a woman's menstrual cycle. Some people with MS find that walking problems are worse after meals, and so prefer to exercise earlier in the day, such as before breakfast.
- Cooling down before exercise. The body can lose heat in four ways: conduction (touching a cooler object), convection (increasing air/water flow over the skin), radiation (constantly emitting heat like a radiator) and evaporation (sweating). People with MS often find that they don't sweat as much as they used to, even on hot days, and so rely more on conduction and convection to cool down. Contact with cool, moving water is the quickest way of losing body heat. Learn to love cool showers or baths! Although the body will soon adapt to the shock, you can ease yourself into it by dropping the

temperature of the shower and increasing the time spent under it over a number of days or weeks. Don't be surprised if you find you need to pee soon after the shower! You could also try drinking 1–2 cups of slushed ice before exercise.

- Cooling during exercise. There are numerous body-cooling devices ('coolwear'), several of which have been designed specifically for people with MS. They are generally effective, but can be bulky and expensive. The most affordable ones use ice pouches carried next to the skin in vests, scarves or hats. Other devices involve water sprays that help increase evaporation heat loss, or motorised cooling (such as vests).

- Many people with MS enjoy exercising in water. Not only do swimming and hydrotherapy (exercising in water), for example, allow exercise at various intensities without overheating quickly, the water physically supports those with greater disability while they exercise. If you are fortunate enough to have access, you could also try outdoor swimming in lakes or the sea at certain times of the year (local outdoor swimming clubs will be able to help): a number of studies have shown that such 'wild' swimming is particularly good for mental and physical health.

You can do more if you exercise at different times of the day or year in different places, or cool down before, during and after exercise

- Cooling after exercise. Body temperature can remain increased for some time after finishing exercise, and active cooling (e.g. cold showers or baths, slushed ice, coolwear, cooling bed mattresses) can help recovery.

Other exercise aids

Feel free to buy a whole load of new kit when you start the exercise program, but it's really not necessary. Some people with MS find that paying for expensive gym membership motivates them to exercise, while others take great pleasure in exercising for free, using no special equipment. Whatever works for you!

You don't need lots of expensive equipment to exercise

Certain bits of exercise kit are useful for people with MS. For example, flippers compensate for a weak leg-kick when swimming. Walking poles help balance and work the upper body when walking. Weight machines are generally safer when learning how to lift weights correctly. Heart rate monitors can help you to exercise at a certain intensity (but can be inaccurate in people with MS). Electric bikes? A revelation!

Straight away, you can start to think about some exercise goals based around these devices: why not aim to build strength, stamina and balance so that you can stop using them so much (if at all) during exercise? Aim to swim a length, legs only/no flippers, for example. Or aim to lift free weights or your bodyweight. Or aim to listen to the body and how hard it's exercising. Or reduce the amount you use the electric motor when cycling.

Of course, there are specific physical aids that people with MS may need to use in order to exercise, in addition to the cooling devices described above. For example, splints, sticks and functional electrical stimulation (FES) devices may help with balance and extend range when starting to exercise. Again, these provide other exercise goals: why not train the body and mind to stop using these during exercise? And then extend these gains into not using them in everyday life?

Keeping a daily record of exercise and the goals reached is a powerful motivational tool for keeping up a regular exercise routine

Whatever you decide, probably the cheapest and most motivational exercise aid is a daily record of all the exercise you do and all the goals you've set. People with MS commonly perceive that their illness gets worse over time. Keeping a log can be invaluable in reminding you that this is not always the case. Remember two years ago when you were overweight and eating poorly, smoking, stressed and unfit—and you were diagnosed with

MS? Well, look at what you've achieved since then: feels pretty good to have run your first 5k, or walked your daughter down the aisle, doesn't it?

Ground covered

Exercise is a core pillar of the OMS lifestyle. It's never too late to start exercising. Some exercise is better than none at all. Exercise will not make MS worse: quite the opposite. It slows the effects of the illness. It improves physical and mental health, and quality of life. Find a way of incorporating different exercises that you enjoy into your life. Aim for 'functional' fitness, so that you can stay healthy and carry on living life independently. But remember the need to find the balance between exercising enough to see the benefits, but not so much that your health suffers.

It can be hard to get into the habit of exercising, but the benefits are worth it. Have a chat with yourself about what barriers are stopping you exercising, and how you can overcome these; have a chat with friends, family and other people about how they can help you overcome any barriers. Try building regular exercise into your life using the '5 Cs' approach: commit, check, change slowly but often, be consistent, and care for yourself.

Acknowledgement

I would like to thank Professor Giselle Petzinger, MD, a movement disorders specialist at the Keck School of Medicine, University of Southern California, and UK psychotherapist Ms Jo Woods for their comments and suggestions on earlier drafts of this chapter.

My Story: Claes Nermark

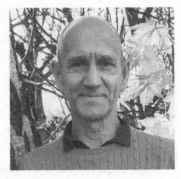

It was 20 May 2010: 'I think you should call an ambulance and come in right now!' That was the response I got when I called the hospital information service. It had been a very busy period during which I was transition-ing from a job at a fitness club to being manager at a new start-up in holistic health. Driving home that afternoon I had begun to experience very noticeable double vision.

As I had been diagnosed with a stroke in 2002 after a period of optic neuritis, my wife Malin persuaded me to make that call. She drove me to the hospital immediately. Two days, an MRI scan and a lumbar puncture later, I was diagnosed with MS. As I had no knowledge of the disease, I was never really scared after receiving the news. I was very focused on getting well enough to get back to my exciting new job. Malin, on the other hand, having strong memories of her grandmother in a wheelchair due to MS, took on all the worrying, and ordered a lot of books about MS.

Luckily, one of the books was *Overcoming Multiple Sclerosis* with its 7 step guide to recovery, a program for healing MS backed up with tons of research. Compared with the 'disease-modifying drugs is your only option' message I got from my neurologist, it seemed almost too good to be true. Having a strong belief in the body's capacity to heal, I wholeheartedly threw myself into the OMS Program on top of other healing modalities that Malin had read about in other books. I started out well with lots of hope and enthusiasm but soon hit a bit of a bumpy patch.

Being a trained physical education teacher and a fitness instruc-tor, exercise and movement were a vital part of my life. The first six months were tough as my double vision got worse every time my body temperature increased during workouts. I had to change to walking, swimming, yoga and qi gong to keep active. When my vision was back to normal I gradually and carefully increased the intensity of my fitness routines and returned to my previous fitness levels.

In July 2013 I participated together with Malin in the first one-week residential OMS retreat in England with 35 people with MS, as well as a few partners. All came to the retreat with one common goal: overcoming MS. Apart from making friends for life, the experience deepened my understanding of the OMS Program and it has served as a roadmap for going forward ever since.

I had some relapses and other symptoms during the first three years after starting out on the Program, but as they got milder as well as less frequent, I decided to gear up on my exercise to find out if my recovery could stand a true endurance challenge. In the summer of 2013 I enrolled in and completed the 300 kilometre bike race called 'Vättern runt', which is a bike ride around the second largest lake in Sweden. I did this without symptoms or other problems (apart from a sore bottom). This was when Malin told me what the abbreviation MS really was to me—Mental Strength!

I've now been relapse-free for seven years and the road ahead is filled with hope and positivity. I work full-time as a wellness manager for a global company, a role that includes quite a bit of travelling. I conduct weekly yoga and fitness classes. Other challenges I've completed include a 30-kilometre cross-country run and an Olympic Triathlon (consisting of a 1500-metre open-water swim, a 40-kilometre bike ride and a 10-kilometre run). Expressing gratitude is a vital part of my meditations and, to me, being an OMSer equals being an Outstanding Mover and Shaker.

6

Meditation, mindfulness and the mind-body connection

Associate Professor Craig Hassed

I've taken control of being me!

Sue Allaway, Torquay, UK, OMSer

For better or worse, the mind is a powerful influence on our mental and physical health and the lifestyle we lead. It can work for us or against us. It can generate stress out of thin air or help us to be at peace even in the most adverse situations. It can drive the healthy changes that we want to make in our lives or serve as a roadblock to progress. It can operate in mysterious and bewildering ways like a GPS taking us totally in the wrong direction. But with care and attention, we can learn how the mind works and direct it to where we want to go. For these and other reasons, we need to learn more about the mind and how to use it well, and that is where meditation and mindfulness come in.

In this chapter we are going to consider what stress is, when it is useful and when it's not, and how the mind and body are so intimately connected. We will then explore how mindfulness and meditation can contribute to our mental and physical wellbeing as well as help with coping with a chronic condition like MS.

Mental health and MS are intimately related

Stress, poor mental health and physical health problems are closely related. It is really a two-way street—one leads to the other and vice versa. Thus, in susceptible people one's mental and emotional state can trigger or accelerate the development and progression of chronic conditions such as MS. By the same token, MS can cause or exacerbate stress and mental health problems such as depression for a range of reasons, including the negative impact that MS can have on a person's life, and also its impact as an inflammatory condition on the brain.

Understanding the relationship between mind and body and how stress affects them will help us to understand why it is worth practising mindfulness, so let's take that little detour now.

Stress and poor mental health are intimately connected to physical health

What is the stress response and does it have an upside?

Stress is a commonly used term that covers a wide range of human experiences. Some describe it as a 'perceived inability to cope' or when 'demands exceed means'. It is used to describe the physical effects associated with anxiety or fear, including muscle tension, tremulousness, clamminess and rapid heartbeat. These physical effects, especially when chronic, can lead to tiredness and many other symptoms. Stress is also a word used to refer to psychological, emotional and existential states such as confusion, distractibility, forgetfulness, worry, fear, anger, frustration, aimlessness, despondency and depression, although stress and depression are quite different conditions.

The stress response, otherwise known as the 'fight or flight response', is a natural, necessary and appropriate physiological response to an exceptional situation. For example, in the present moment if you are about to be attacked by a tiger, or to be run over by a truck, then you need to respond quickly to either *fight* off the danger or *fly* out of the way. A little turbocharge button in your brain (the amygdala) goes off. If you were paying attention to your body when it was activating the fight or flight response, you would notice the adrenaline, cortisol and other chemicals having a very rapid effect with the following manifestations:

- the circulation becomes 'hyper-dynamic' (increased heart-rate, blood pressure)
- blood drains from the skin (going pale) and gastrointestinal tract (dry mouth, gut stops working) so that the blood can be sent to the muscles
- the muscles gear up for action
- fuels (sugars and fats) are pumped rapidly into the bloodstream
- all of a sudden we feel hungry for air because we need oxygen to burn the fuel and we need to exhale carbon dioxide (our exhaust system)
- the engine is revving fast (metabolic rate going up), leaving us feeling hot
- we sweat (to keep ourselves cool while we exert ourselves)
- the blood gets thick and sticky ready to clot rapidly in order to stop potential bleeding if we get injured (it's 'blood curdling')
- the body pumps out inflammatory chemicals to mobilise tissue repair and rapidly activate our immune system to fight off potential infections in case we get injured.

This sounds like anxiety, but it's not. It's activation, and if we're lucky it will be the difference between life and death. This activation or stress response, based on a clearly perceived present moment threat, is meant to be good for our health, not bad for our health. It is encoded into our genes, brain and physiology to preserve life by allowing the body to respond rapidly and decisively to dangerous situations. For a short period of time our defences will be on high alert and we will be faster, stronger and have more endurance than we normally have. When the situation is over the body will return to rest if the mind leaves the event in the past and moves on by re-engaging with what is happening now—like sitting around a campfire with friends and family, eating a meal, and sharing yarns about nearly getting caught by a tiger.

The replaying of the past event in the mind or anticipating it again in the future, however, can reproduce the stress response even though, in reality, we may be in a completely stress-free environment. If you've ever been awake at 3 a.m. worrying over something then you will know what that feels like. Present moment reality may be as comfortable as life can get—soft mattress and pillow, warm blankets and quiet room—and yet the mind can be projecting 1001 'what ifs' and 'maybes' about the future or replaying myriad things from the past (generally with embellishments).

If we are not mindful, we can spend the whole night fighting with the phantoms of our very fertile imaginations by mistaking imagination to be real, in which case the body faithfully translates it into the fight or flight response, as if there was a phantom or tiger in the room. But that is not a turbocharge of energy—we have other names for it like stress or anxiety. When people say, 'stress is bad for our health', it's this unnecessary activation that is being spoken of.

There will of course be challenges in our lives that do need attention, but when the moment comes to deal with a challenge or decision, then we give it our full and undivided attention. Once it is done, we leave it behind and move on to the next thing, whether it is another challenge or decision, or whether it is just a mundane task like making ourselves a cup of tea with almond milk in it.

If we are mindful, it is relatively easy to tell the difference between imagination and reality. To see what is meant by that, do an experiment now. Imagine a tiger. Look at that imaginary tiger. Are you afraid that the tiger you have just imagined is actually going to attack you? Probably not. Why not? Because you can see it is only in your imagination therefore it has no capacity to activate the stress response. But when we are catastrophising about some hypothetical event in the future, or having an imaginary argument with someone in our heads, or replaying something we regret from the past, do we also realise that too is only in our imagination? If we don't, then it has great power to needlessly activate the stress response, putting a lot of wear and tear on the body and strain on the mind, and distracts us from the actual life we are leading. If we do realise it is in our imagination, then we may be able to ground ourselves back in present-moment reality through the senses by feeling the pillow under our cheek, the breath going in and out of our nose, feeling the teabag we are jiggling in the teacup, paying attention to the road if we are driving, or listening closely to the person speaking to us. This is what is meant by coming to our senses. It is simple but profoundly beneficial for mind and body.

All things have their place and in their proper place all things can be useful; this goes for stress also, but only if used intelligently. Not only can the appropriate 'fight or flight response' help us to adapt to threatening situations but it can be a useful motivation to shift us out of inertia and procrastination and improve performance.

It has another use also. Emotional and mental pain are similar to physical pain in that they're there for a reason. If we have a broken leg we know that the physical pain is trying to give us some very useful information, albeit unpleasant, about which part of the body is hurt and in need of support and healing. If appropriate attention is given to the injured part, healing takes place and wholeness and strength are restored.

So it is with mental and emotional pain. If we just block out or numb the pain with some strong pain-killer, without due care for the injured part, then we may appear better off but we continue to do damage to ourselves. Many of our ways of dealing with stress are like this. We try and block out or react to the stress with aggression, denial, drugs or distraction, but these give only the appearance of comfort or temporary relief. The problem is likely to get compounded and more deeply entrenched unless we pay attention to the stress, in which case we have the opportunity to recognise its source (e.g. unhelpful patterns of thought, worry, self-criticism) and do something more constructive. So, although stress is not pleasant or desirable in itself, it can be used constructively.

What is the role of perception in stress?

The body does what the mind, consciously or unconsciously, tells it to do. If we imagine a rope to be a snake, the body will react to what we perceive, not the reality. Even events that are actually happening may or may not cause stress depending on what the mind thinks about them. One person seeing a mouse running through the kitchen sees a mouse, another sees a monster and another, perhaps a five-year-old, sees a potential pet. It's not the mouse that determines that; it is ourselves and what we project onto situations.

Thus, the mind has the key role of eliciting the stress response through its functions of perception, cognition, interpretation and conditioning. Personality and healthy and unhealthy patterns of behaviour are inherited to some extent but they are also learned. Learned patterns of coping and personality styles are possibly more important than a situation itself in determining how much stress we experience.

Events are just events. It is our thinking that interprets them as a stressor, threat, opportunity or something of interest or disinterest. Studies on people living with MS have shown that those who experience 'stressful' life events but have a positive view of stress actually have a reduced number of relapses, whereas people with MS who view stress in a negative way have a significantly increased number of relapses if stressful events happen in their life. 'But', you might say, 'that doesn't make sense.'

Our responses to stress can be positive or negative; the actual consequences are quite different depending on the response

It has much to do with how we label and think about events. If we drop the word 'stressful' from life events and use the word 'challenging' instead, it changes our perception of the situation. An event can certainly be challenging, like losing a job or receiving a diagnosis of MS, but the way we see and respond to it matters enormously. One person sees a disaster, gets lost in rumination, and projects into and starts living in a mental future that may or may not even happen. This can certainly lead to post-traumatic stress. Another person who has the same thing happen experiences the event but, although it may hurt like hell, sees it as a major challenge through which they can learn about themselves, rethink what really matters in life and find reserves of strength that may have been lying dormant. Such a person has the potential for post-traumatic growth.

None of this trivialises the challenging things that can happen to us in life but it reminds us of what Viktor Frankl called the last of human freedoms, which was 'to choose one's attitude in any given set of circumstances, to choose one's own way'. This he discovered for himself while being held prisoner in the Nazi concentration camps.

Acknowledging this freedom empowers us to be more proactive and understand ourselves better by taking conscious charge of our responses. Any response to stress that merely apportions blame to the environment and external events will be of very limited value as it ignores the most important element in the process: the person responding to the environment. But we must be careful, in acknowledging the role we play in generating our own stress, not to get caught in self-blame. That is another commonly taken wrong turn that leads to nowhere useful. Responsibility is much more about fostering a healthy 'ability to respond' than it is about blame or recrimination.

Taking a wrong turn—how does stress affect health?

If we take a wrong turn and keep going down the road that leads to stress (and who hasn't done that?), then the unhelpful, unmindful kind of chronic stress described above can have many negative impacts on our physical and mental health. These are direct effects of stress on the body, but also indirect effects, because our state of mind is so important in influencing the healthy and unhealthy choices we make. So, here is a little of the bad news before we look at the good news.

Direct effects: the mind–body connection

The unnecessary and excessive switching on of the stress response, though common, is not healthy; nor does it help us to cope with demands. In fact, it does quite the opposite. When the mind is agitated and unfocused we can, and usually do, become over-whelmed with imaginings, projections, negative self-talk and anticipation, which are all given a reality that they do not deserve. The long-term effect of this is wear and tear on the body called *allostatic load*. There is a lot of allostatic load in stress, anxiety and depression. It's like using the car we have been given and flogging it so that its parts wear out faster. The cumulative effects can accelerate ageing and the progression of chronic illnesses, including autoimmune conditions.

It does this in no small part because of the chronic production of these inflammatory chemicals with fancy names like cytokines and interleukins. They are great when we are wrestling a tiger, but not so useful when we are producing them day in day out in excess of what is required. The short-term burst of immunity when fighting the imaginary tigers soon turns into what is called *immune dysregulation*. What that means is that we have less defence against colds, flus and other infections and we suffer more inflammation. It's the worst of both worlds. The immune system doesn't do what we want it to do (protect us from pathogens) and it does more of what we don't want it to do (cause inflammation and attack our own bodies as if they were foreign invaders).

What that means for MS is that increased inflammation leads to more lesions, more relapses and more progression, unless we learn how to recognise the unnecessary activation of the stress response and to switch it off. The best way to do that, from a mindfulness perspective, is to come back to the present moment: if you realise that the stress was due to your mind getting a bit ahead of itself, the response will switch itself off. Dealing with 'what is' is a lot easier than dealing with the endless 'what ifs' that the mind can come up with.

Happily, learning to be more mindful and meditating on a regular basis can help to reverse these effects.

Indirect effects: lifestyle choices and relationships

Apart from the direct mind–body effects described above, when needlessly over-activating the stress response, we also feel awful emotionally, our quality of life dives, and it is hard to connect meaningfully with the life we are leading and the people we are with.

The indirect negative effects of stress on our mental and physical health are because they also influence the lifestyle choices we make. If, for example, we smoke, it is harder to get off the cigarettes, or if we are trying to stop smoking, the stress can undermine our resolve and strength to stay off them. The same goes for any addiction, including excessive alcohol or drug use.

Likewise, if we don't feel happy in ourselves, we are also more likely to reach for the habitual and comfort foods that might give us momentary pleasure but cause long-term health problems, especially for a condition like MS. It can also negatively affect our readiness to exercise, ability to sleep well and the quality of our relationships. All of this can seriously impact the physical health and progression of MS.

This all adds up to the fact that the mind is the most centrally important factor in our road to good health. The mind is like the driver of the car. To drive well, navigate effectively, avoid accidents and look after the car, the driver's skill, attention to the road and temperament are all important.

Getting back on track—managing stress more mindfully

Well, you've had the bad news. The good news is that if we have taken a wrong turn down the road to stress. we can turn things around and get back onto either the scenic route or the main highway of life if we want to take the shortest route to where we want to go. All these negative effects mentioned above are reversible if we practise switching off the stress response when we don't need it. The best way to do that is by being mindful of the present moment and the best way to be more present is by practising meditation regularly.

Practising meditation by itself isn't enough for an illness to just go away, but it does mean that we can help the body to do the healing it wants to do by taking the unnecessary or excess stress off the body, and we can also make more conscious lifestyle choices. Training the mind, dealing with stress and having a supportive community of like-minded people are the first things to get right because they make all the other lifestyle choices so much easier.

Practising mindfulness meditation regularly is a very effective way of managing stress

What does it mean to be mindful?

We have already hinted at what it means to be unmindful—distracted, inattentive, disengaged and reactive. Being mindful is pretty much the opposite of that—in other words: present, aware, accepting and engaged. It really involves training attention and attitude.

Being able to give our attention to the things we want to or need to give attention to also helps us to not allocate our attention to unhelpful things like worry, rumination, catastrophising and negative self-talk. Being able to be more aware in the moment allows us to understand ourselves better rather than living life on automatic pilot. If we are going to be less and less interested in the tendency to worry or ruminate, then what do we get interested in instead? Perhaps our life's journey might become the focus of our attention, from the mundane moments to the most profound.

People get very focused on the attention side of the mindfulness equation, but attitude matters as much as attention, perhaps even more so. The mindful attitude means practising being less and less judgemental, reactive, critical and angry and instead practising being more open, accepting, non-reactive, kind and compassionate. To realise how important attitude is, just consider the effect that a negative or critical attitude has when you are having thoughts (e.g. worry) and feelings (e.g. anxiety) that you don't want to have. The more reactive to them you are, the more the attention goes to them and the stronger and more influential they become. We get the exact opposite of what we intend—instead of being free of them we get caught up in them. Notice that. Learn from it. Our experiences will have tried thousands and thousands of times to teach us that lesson, but we rarely stop long enough to notice the lesson. If a judgemental or critical attitude leads in one direction, where does a less judgmental and critical attitude lead? The opposite direction, of course.

Mindfulness may be simple but it's not easy

These changes in attention and attitude take time but, even when we think we are getting nowhere, every time we practise we are taking a step in the right direction. We are rewiring our brain for better attention and a gentler attitude. Sooner or later it will start to make itself evident in our lives. sometimes, strangely, without us hardly noticing.

Having read this you are probably coming to the conclusion that mindfulness is pretty simple, which it is, but it's not easy.

How can mindfulness help promote better mental health?
When we learn to be more mindful and less caught in repetitive patterns of worry and rumination, it has the effect of lessening anxiety and depression, the two most common conditions that negatively impact mental health. There are other benefits as well, such as lessening the impact of anger or resentment. Replacing these conditions is a growing sense of being able to be present in our life and to savour the moment and enjoy the simple pleasures that are there if we care to look. It's like we start to enjoy the journey of life all over again with less of the anxious preoccupation about getting to the destination.

How do we cultivate mindfulness in our lives?
As mindfulness is both a form of meditation and a way of living, there are two main ways to practise being mindful in our lives: the formal and informal practices. The formal practice is also called mindfulness meditation, where we sit down and do nothing other than be mindful for a period of time, whether that is a short time (e.g. 30 seconds) or a longer time (e.g. 30 minutes). The aim of practising meditation, however, is not to be mindful for a few

minutes and then just go back to an unmindful life on automatic pilot. The aim is to live more mindfully for the full 24 hours of the day. To put it another way, you practise some mindfulness meditation before you get into the car so that you can then drive with more awareness and clarity for the whole of your journey.

The formal practice (meditation)

There are plenty of good mindfulness resources and apps around that can help guide you through meditation. These can be very useful, especially early on in your meditation journey. Guided practices are a little like putting training wheels on a bike—they help us not to fall off. But, just as the aim is not to spend our whole life riding bikes with training wheels, the ultimate aim is not to need external guidance for meditation practice. Over time it is best to develop our own internal ability to be mindful. Having the training wheels on (guidance) generally makes meditation easier and more pleasant and taking off the training wheels (practising by ourselves) generally is more challenging because we fall off the bike more (our mind wanders, we get irritated with ourselves, we fight with our thoughts and feelings).

Therefore, many people assume that guided practice is best, but if you look at it from a different perspective—which situation will train your balance better, training wheels on or training wheels off? Ultimately, the unguided practice is the best.

Preparation

It is often easier to practise the exercise in a quiet place without interruptions but this is not always possible. Noise need not preclude the practice at all; but we may notice that in a stimulating environment distractibility and the activity of the mind are increased greatly, so we just have to practise not judging and bringing the attention back more frequently than would otherwise be the case.

It is recommended that the exercise be practised for at least five minutes twice daily (before breakfast and dinner are good times) and at other times during the day if needed. These other times could be only for a minute each, or even a few seconds, just to help break the build-up of tension throughout the day. Over time, according to your level of motivation, you can build up the time to 10, 15, 20 or even 30 minutes twice a day.

While practising this exercise, there is no need to 'try' or put in effort, except in so far as we remember to not judge ourselves and to bring the attention back when it wanders off. Don't be perturbed if mental activity continues throughout; that does not necessarily mean that the exercise is not beneficial. The important thing is to practise 'letting go', or not feeding the activity with attention, because it is the attention that gives this distracted thinking its power. Allow each phase of the exercise to occur effortlessly. Paradoxically, trying to make an experience happen, like peace or an empty mind, tends to increase tension and mental activity. The practice is very simple; in short it is a matter of resting the attention on something and being uninterested in everything else.

Position
Sit in an upright, balanced but relaxed position with the back and neck straight and held without any tension, and with the hands resting on the lap. Outside of practising at night in bed, if the position is too comfortable it will become an exercise in going to sleep, rather than waking up and being aware. Conversely, if the body is uncomfortable or unbalanced, this too can have a distracting effect on the mind. Some choose to practise the exercise lying down. This can also be satisfactory if the back is straight and the body symmetrically positioned although many people find this position too readily leads to sleep, which might be useful in the middle of the night but is not generally useful during the day. The relaxation of sleep is not the same as the restful awareness of mindfulness.

Body scan
Adopt the position as above. Let the eyes gently close and begin the exercise. We are going to use the sense of touch to help the

mind to be in the present moment because the body is already and always present—it is the mind that is often absent. So, become aware of the body's posture. Notice its presence in the room, here and now. Just rest in that. If thoughts, attitudes or feelings arise, let them come and pass as they will without having to do anything about them or even thinking they shouldn't be there.

Let the body feel its full weight and fall still. Notice the sensation of the clothes or the air on the skin, the body's weight on the chair or the feet on the floor. If you are happy to, allow the attention to rest for a while with one particular part of the body at a time—for example, the feet—then the legs, stomach, chest, hands, arms, shoulders and neck, and then the head.

Breathing
Take a couple of deeper breaths, slowly let them out, and with the out-breath let any muscle tension fall away. Then let the breathing fall into its own natural rhythm, gentle and smooth, without interfering or controlling it in any particular way. The body knows how to breathe so just let it. Observe and feel the breath. Rest the attention where the air enters and leaves the body. During this or any other stage of the exercise, distracting thoughts and feelings may come into the mind. Just practise watching them like images on a movie screen, remembering that the mind is playing a movie. Or practise watching them like passing trains of thought—there is no need to stop them, but just practise standing on the railway platform without getting on the trains. Even if you try and stop these thoughts coming into mind, notice the effect that has. Be curious. Your experience will teach you what works and what doesn't. Let thoughts be observed and let them pass again, allowing the attention to gently return to an awareness of the breath. We are not able to necessarily stop the thoughts and daydreams, but we can practise standing back, observing, detaching and letting go of them. This includes the happy daydreams as well as the unhappy ones. We are practising waking up out of daydreams and becoming aware in the present; that is presence of mind, not absent-mindedness.

Listening
Now, if you are happy to, just listen to all the sounds you can hear around you. Let them be received by the ears as they come and go. Listen as far into the distance as you can. There is no need to think about where the sounds come from or where they go to, what they mean or anything else. Just listen and rest, once again letting thoughts and feelings pass as they arise. Choose to direct the listening away from any chatter or noise in the mind and reconnect it with the real sounds, even if your mind is talking with itself about mindfulness meditation and how it's going. At the completion of this phase take a deep breath in and out, gently open the eyes and, when ready, mindfully move into the activities that await you.

The most important thing about meditation is to practise regularly

The importance of practice
Some people feel like they fail at meditation, mostly because they are unable to stop the thoughts or let go of all the tensions. There is no such thing as failing the exercise. There is no pressure to relax or to make the mind go blank. If it arises, we can learn to be more comfortable with discomfort such as stress, anger or fear. We can learn to worry less about trying not to worry. We practise training attention and attitude—practise gently bringing the attention back and being non-judgemental and self-compassionate.

Mindfulness will make us more aware of what is going on, warts and all. That's a sign of it working. It is more a matter of observing whatever is going on with less and less attitude to it. Success and failure are simply part of the thinking going on in the mind that needs to be let go of. The important thing is to practise these techniques and let the process mature over time. If the mind remains active don't worry, just practise not getting caught up with the activity. While noting it, and the sorts of things that tend to repeat, learn to be uninterested in it. Learn to be less moved by it. Over time this takes a lot of the force out of these thoughts and therefore gives us a significant level of freedom from them.

The informal practice (daily life)

As previously mentioned, the aim of mindfulness meditation is not to have a time-out in a hellish day, it is to help us to be more mindful in daily life, whether communicating, eating, driving, resting, walking or doing anything else. If we are living unmindfully, the journey becomes a blur. We not only miss the life we are living but, among other things, we also miss the opportunity to learn, savour or make more conscious choices in life. The costs are significant but often unrecognised.

So, how do we become more mindful in daily life? It's simple really. We just need to come to our senses. When our attention is connected to the senses (seeing, hearing, feeling, tasting or smelling), the default circuits associated with daydreaming, worry or rumination are switched off and attention circuits are switched on. We are, as they say, in touch with reality. Because we are no longer unconsciously consumed by our daydreams, worries or ruminations, the mind can perceive things a little more clearly in accord with what is really happening. It gives us the chance to make better decisions and respond more rationally—that's what is meant by the term 'coming to our senses'.

In a practical sense, when walking through the park, just feel the movement of the body, hear the sound of the birds, see the colours of the flowers or smell the scent in the air. When driving your car, look at the road. When slicing the vegetables, feel the knife in your hand and look at the thing you are slicing. When you are with your doctor, look at them and listen to what they are saying. The thing about living mindfully in daily life is that it is not hard work, but it does require practice. When mindful we are constantly giving the mind a rest from all the things that are superfluous and that it doesn't need to be thinking about in that moment.

Just one other point that may save a little confusion and frustration. When you are mindful, you don't need to practise mindfulness because you're mindful already. At such times we're not thinking about ourselves, we are just living in the moment. When the mind is away with the birds, running down rabbit holes or off in its own little world of rumination, that's when we need to practise mindfulness by coming back to the present moment through the senses. Thinking about whether or not we are paying attention is not the same as actually paying attention—it's thinking pretending to be useful. It's as big a distraction as any other distraction.

Urge surfing

Let's just imagine that as you journey home along the coast road you notice a beautiful beach with waves rolling in, so you think it might be good to stop for a while, go for a paddle in the water and cool off. While there you decide to learn how to go 'urge surfing'.

Changing habits isn't easy. Stopping smoking or eating foods that are unhealthy for us or diving back into worry or rumination, for example, isn't easy. To make the lifestyle changes we want to make we need to learn to deal with the cravings and urges to go back to our old patterns of behaviour. The habitual way is to suppress or fight these urges, but this comes at a cost as far as stress and emotional energy are concerned. Sooner or later, when our guard is down or we are in a vulnerable moment, the vast majority of us go for the cigarette packet, the comfort food or the worry, even though there is another part of us trying to pull us back. Having done the unhealthy thing, the next unmindful thing that we generally do is to launch into self-criticism and negative self-talk about what a terrible person we must be. It's doubly stressful, time wasting and very demotivating.

To make healthy changes, we need to learn to 'surf' rather than 'fight' the urge to smoke, eat unhealthy food, worry or do anything else for that matter. When an urge arises it's like a wave. If we struggle against it, we will probably be swamped by it. Understandably, we think we need to control the urge rather than learning how not to be controlled by it. From a mindfulness perspective, what we can do instead is to ride the urge like a wave—let the wave pick us up and float on the surface of it, like surfers do. This urge, like every other urge we have ever had in our lives, rises and then subsides again. Some urges, like waves, are bigger than others, but we can learn to ride them all.

On a practical level, what this means is that there's no need to do anything other than practise observing and standing back from the urge without getting involved in it. That means not getting attached to it, reacting to it or even thinking it shouldn't be there. When we react to it, we get drawn into it, give it our energy and then it has the power to influence us. When we sit and practise mindfulness meditation, or when we go about being mindful in our day-to-day life, we will notice urges, emotions and impulses coming and going all the time. In fact, meditation often makes us more aware of them but we can welcome that because it gives us the chance to practise urge surfing. It's a waste of time and effort wishing they weren't there, because they already are, but we can practise letting them flow in and through. Just noticing the urge in a 'matter of fact' kind of way, noticing if the mind starts to imagine the future ('how happy I would be if I could . . .'), noticing the physical response (longing or tensing up) and noticing where the attention goes (meditating on an imaginary me having the imaginary thing). Patiently, non-judgementally and gently, practise by escorting the attention back to the body or breath or whatever else we're practising being mindful of.

Mindfulness meditation helps us to better manage the peaks and troughs of life

There's no need to wonder when urges will stop coming because that's also about the future. Mindfulness is only about ever working in the moment now. We don't have to give something up for some dim, dark, deprived future stretching out forever. We are likely to get despondent ruminating about that; we only need to let it go now. Every moment we practise letting the urges come and go, we get better at surfing. It takes practice, patience and a considerable amount of self-compassion, but over time the urges come and go more and more easily until they create less and less disturbance and distraction on the way through.

Are we there yet?

The following slightly cryptic message was once noticed on a desk calendar: 'When you finally get *there* you realise there is no *there*'. Well, if there is no *there*, there must only be *here*. Is the journey of mindfulness really about going somewhere else, or is it really about coming back to where we already are? Are we trying to learn something new and foreign to us, or merely reacquainting ourselves with that sense of *being* within us—something so familiar that we may have long forgotten it since the simplicity and innocence of childhood? Who knows? We have to discover this for ourselves. Nobody else can take our journey for us, but the journey within is the most interesting and surprising journey we can take.

Ground covered

We have covered a lot of ground in this chapter. Starting off from the 'crossroads of bewildering choices', we chose the meandering path leading to 'understanding the influence of the mind', went past the wrong turn leading to 'stress', and followed the signposts of 'clear perception' and 'conscious choices' that directed us to the mindfulness superhighway. Along the way, we stopped off for a mindful rest and a bit of urge surfing. All we need to do now is to stay on the highway and it will take us all the way to the end of our journey, the twin towns of 'peace of mind' and 'self-discovery'. I'll see you there!

My Story:
Dr Véronique Gauthier

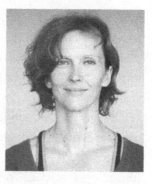

I was diagnosed with RRMS in 2000. At the time I was lecturing at University College Dublin while completing my PhD thesis. I was smoking 30 cigarettes a day, but I was also addicted to the gym—especially spinning and step aerobics. I worked hard, played hard and slept very little. That was the perfect life, or so I thought. Then one day, in a step aerobics class, I completely lost control of my right foot. Although I recovered within an hour, I kept having weird sensations in my legs. Shortly afterwards, my vision went blurry while playing squash.

As symptoms accumulated over the following months, I thought it might be a good idea to 'slow down a bit'. Yoga was becoming popular in Dublin so I decided to give it a try, although, to be honest, I thought it would be boring. It turned out to be love at the first try. The first class I attended was an ashtanga class. For a full hour, we stretched, balanced, strengthened and, most importantly, we focused on the breath. It must have been the first time that I paid attention to my breath for so long and it felt really good! The 'ujjayi' breath, in which you inhale and exhale through the nose while slightly contracting the throat, became my new addiction.

Although the first years after diagnosis were really tough, practising yoga helped me a lot. In fact, it helped me so much that in 2009 I decided to train as a yoga teacher because I wanted to share the benefits of yoga with other people living with MS. Thanks to yoga, I became aware of how the body affects the mind, and vice versa. I also discovered tools, such as yoga poses, breathing techniques and meditations, to restore balance in my life.

By the time I discovered the *Overcoming Multiple Sclerosis* book in 2012, I was an ex-smoker, mainly vegetarian, qualified yoga teacher. I was starting to feel better but still experienced relapses once or twice a year. With hindsight, I now know that my diet was wrong—I was eating too much *camembert*—and that I was deficient in vitamin D3. But I was also missing a sense of direction and a community. When I read Professor Jelinek's book, I felt relieved and empowered. Relieved because I was on the right track. Empowered because the book explained what I should do to overcome MS.

As I gradually became more engaged with OMS, first joining the forum and then becoming a facilitator, I found 'my' community. After the mind–body connection, I discovered the healing power of the human connection. On 4 February 2020 I celebrated twenty years of living with MS. I now work full-time from my beautiful home in southern Portugal. Besides yoga I do strengthening exercises and swim in the ocean regularly. Right now I'm also training for my first marathon. I have no doubt that I would never have been able to do this without yoga and the OMS Program.

7

Medication

Dr Jonathan White

> The ideal situation is when you can work in partnership with your doctor, exploring both lifestyle and pharmaceutical options.
>
> *Fiona Shultz, Geelong, Australia, OMSer*

The use of medication where appropriate in the treatment of MS is one of the key steps of the OMS Program. People with MS should have a clear understanding of the whole topic of using medications to assist in the management of the disease, to empower them to make what can be very significant and life-changing decisions. It is important for anyone considering embarking on drug treatment to have access to relevant, impartial information, and to take the time to consider all options. It is equally important to acknowledge that for some people, medication is simply not the right personal choice, and this should be respected.

Given the pivotal role of lifestyle change in influencing the progression of MS, any choice to use medication should be considered as a potential addition to, not a substitute for, a healthy lifestyle. This is in line with the ever-increasing body of evidence outlined in this book and elsewhere demonstrating that factors in our lifestyle that we can change offer the very real chance for long-term good health and wellbeing while living with MS.

Since the introduction of disease-modifying therapies (DMTs) just over twenty years ago, there has been a rapid evolution towards ever more effective treatments for MS. There are currently more than a dozen drug options available for relapsing remitting MS (RRMS), and treatments for progressive forms of the condition are now also finally becoming available, albeit at a much slower rate (Figure 7.1). Regrettably, MS treatments for those with progressive disease are currently only available to a very specific small cohort of patients, owing to budgetary constraints and healthcare resource considerations.

Most authorities now recommend that MS drug treatment should begin as soon as possible after diagnosis, with the aim of reducing disease activity at an early stage, thereby minimising the number of relapses and hopefully also any longer-term disability progression. We reinforce that this also applies to lifestyle management of MS, which should also commence as early as possible after diagnosis.

Controversy remains, however, over how hard to hit the disease at its outset, with some neurologists advocating a gradual escalation in drug treatment, matched to the level of disease activity, thereby reducing potentially unnecessary over-treatment and side effects. On the other side, there are those calling for the newer, more potent 'induction' therapies to be used as first-line treatments, aiming to rapidly suppress the disease. Their rationale is that this provides the best chances of favourable outcomes in the longer term. While the short-to-medium-term data appears to indicate that induction therapy may be the more effective option, we simply

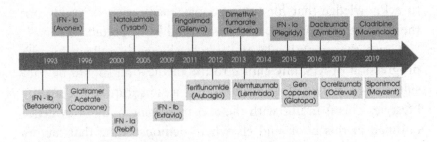

Figure 7.1: The timeline of DMT approval in MS. Source: E. Melamed & M.W. Lee, 'Multiple sclerosis and cancer: The ying-yang effect of disease modifying therapies', *Frontiers in Immunology*, 10, 2954: 2. https://doi.org/10.3389/fimmu.2019.02954

don't yet know the results for those people with MS 20, 30 or even 40 years from the point of diagnosis. Current recommendations, however, frequently discount or do not include the role of significant lifestyle modification at an early stage in the disease process.

It may seem obvious that when choosing a medication for MS, one would simply pick the most effective treatment right from the outset. Unfortunately, the more effective a particular drug is at preventing relapses and disability progression, then generally speaking (apart from the interferons), the greater the side-effect profile and risks, some of which can be very serious. Many people may therefore make a decision to avoid this greater risk by choosing a slightly less potent drug.

Many neurologists aim to treat MS as soon as possible after diagnosis

Up until the mid-1990s, there were no meaningful treatments that could change the course of MS. Yes, short courses of steroids could help a person recover more quickly from individual relapses, but there was very little a doctor could do to slow the almost inevitable march of disability and decline. The best they could do was reassure their patients that in some people, the disease took a more benign course, and to 'hope you were going to fall into that group'.

No doctor goes into medicine to impart news like that to their patients. We are trained to define the problem, and then fix it. We diagnose and we treat. So imagine the great frustration felt on the part of many neurologists in the past, dealing with this relatively poorly understood condition, often without access to tests to provide an accurate diagnosis, and no really useful treatment options. Many felt completely powerless, along with many of those they were trying to help.

When the first drug treatments emerged, one can imagine that the medical community was very willing to accept the limited benefits they could offer, even in the face of the rather narrow and uncertain evidence base, and the often serious side-effect profile. After all, one could argue, the alternative was often much worse.

What then if a patient had a drug treatment option available but felt it wasn't right for them; that they couldn't cope with the side effects, or perhaps considered that changes to their lifestyle might offer an improved quality of life, a reduction in symptoms and just maybe, an improved long-term prognosis? You might be able to sense the frustration on the part of their clinician. After all, they knew better than most the harm that MS could potentially do.

Sometimes there still exists the attitude of 'doctor knows best'. The position of many medical and other health professionals is that, when confronted by something, such as lifestyle modification, of which they have a limited knowledge or understanding, they may simply dismiss it. Either by expressing the age-old maxim 'there is no evidence for any of that', or by making their scepticism clear and by not supporting their patients' wishes for self-management, they may unwittingly take legitimate hope from their patients, and potentially damage the therapeutic relationship. All too often, someone doing all that they can to live and stay well with MS may have their hopes dashed on the rocks of alleged medical science, and made to feel foolish, or even worse, negligent, in their attitude towards their own health.

Lack of time, undoubtedly a very significant factor in today's health services, can prevent some doctors becoming aware of the diverse but increasingly concordant and consistent evidence base underpinning the key tenets of the OMS Program, and the role of lifestyle in the prevention and treatment of many diseases. After all, it is currently thought that up to 80 per cent of disease in developed countries is directly related to our often toxic diet and lifestyle. Only 4 per cent of people in Australia, for example, currently reach the standard of the national dietary guidelines in terms of diet. Globally, more than 50 per cent of people now live with a chronic disease.

Medical school training is also undoubtedly a co-conspirator in all of this. The average medical student receives almost no training in nutrition, and it is still not a mandatory requirement on the curriculum in the vast majority of universities. Fortunately, this is gradually changing, and there are now a number of colleges and societies of 'lifestyle medicine' around the world, pushing hard to ensure that the next generation of doctors is better trained in this critical area than their predecessors.

Unquestionably, medication can be an extremely valuable tool in the treatment of MS, and it is now becoming clear that even the lower-efficacy early treatments (interferon-B and glatiramer) do have an impact on long-term disability progression. One could therefore extrapolate that the more effective treatments will have an even greater long-term benefit, and we can only hope that this proves to be the case. Just think of the potential effectiveness of combining the evidence-based lifestyle modifications with the judicious use of medications. But, as with all lifestyle-related illness, prescribing medication without altering the underlying risks is far less effective than adopting the twofold approach.

Use of a DMT should never be a substitute for adopting a healthy lifestyle; the combination of both lifestyle and medication maximises benefit

What follows is not intended to be an exhaustive resource on all available medication options in the management of MS. This would not only be unwieldy and quickly become outdated, given the pace of drug development, but also wouldn't necessarily serve to give a broader context to the topic. For a summary list of the approved medications at the time of writing, see Chapter 1, 'Understanding multiple sclerosis', by neurologist Dr Brandon Beaber. For more detailed information on specific treatments, the latest edition of Prof Jelinek's book *Overcoming Multiple Sclerosis: The evidence-based 7 step recovery program* is an excellent tool, as are the resources available from many local MS organisations or the OMS website (overcomingms.org).

Steroids (prednisolone, prednisone, methylprednisolone)

The use of steroids in the management of acute MS relapses has been commonplace for many years. They clearly shorten the time to recovery from a relapse. Steroids are most effective when started soon after the onset of new symptoms (up to fourteen days), but have no effect on the level of recovery from a relapse, or on the long-term course of MS. For this reason, and also due to potential side effects, steroids are not always prescribed for every relapse episode but are often reserved for more severe or debilitating symptoms, such as new walking difficulties or those affecting eyesight.

Not all steroids are created equal. When we hear the term 'steroid' we often think of huge bodybuilders, and athletes using drugs to enhance their performance. These are the anabolic steroids. While they do share some properties, they should be considered as very different from corticosteroids used in MS and other inflammatory conditions. 'Steroids' is the commonly short-ened version of the term 'corticosteroids'. Corticosteroids refer to those steroids specifically released from the adrenal glands, which sit on top of the kidneys. Synthetic versions now widely available are many times more potent than the natural forms, and are used in various preparations to treat a range of conditions, such as eczema and psoriasis, asthma, rheumatoid arthritis and systemic lupus erythematosus (SLE).

The benefits of steroids in MS are due to their anti-inflammatory properties. They suppress the immune system by altering the balance of pro- and anti-inflammatory messengers that instruct white blood cells to attack the myelin coating of certain nerve cells. Steroids also make the cell membranes of white blood cells more flexible and less sticky, meaning that they are less able to attach to other cells and damage or destroy them. This mecha-nism is actually very similar to the longer-term effects of following a low-saturated fat diet with omega-3 fatty acid supplementation. MRI scans of the brain show that swelling around individual MS lesions reduces rapidly (often within hours) after a first dose of steroids, allowing improved nerve signal transmission in the affected areas, and a reduction in symptoms.

While they are generally safe when used in short courses of up to seven days, they do come with a significant side-effect profile, especially if used continually in the long term. They can cause weight gain, fluid retention, increased risk of infection, stomach ulcers (they should be prescribed with a tablet, such as omeprazole, to protect the stomach lining), depression or psychosis, muscle weakness, cataracts and osteoporosis. It is for this reason that it is generally recommended that their use is limited to three courses per year, and for no more than three weeks at a time.

A course of steroids is safe and usually improves recovery time from a relapse; oral forms are just as effective as intravenous preparations, and help people with MS avoid hospital admission

The evidence is now clear that a course of oral steroids is just as effective as intravenous, and significantly more convenient for the patient. There is no need to taper the dose after the initial course, and the shorter the course, the safer the treatment.

It is perhaps worth discussing with your doctor the possibility of having a completed prescription on hand at home, particularly early on after diagnosis, so that you can begin a course quickly in the case of a relapse. While starting a course of steroids early in a relapse gives the best results, it may be worth waiting at least 48 hours from the onset of symptoms, as they may not represent a true relapse or require any treatment.

First-generation injectables (interferons and glatiramer)

Introduced into clinical practice in the mid-1990s, the interferon-beta medications (Betaferon or Betaseron, Rebif, Avonex, Plegridy, Extavia) were the first of the DMTs used to treat RRMS. Offering a modest relapse rate reduction of around 30 per cent compared to placebo, they are self-injected, ranging in frequency from alternate days to once weekly.

The interferons appear to alter the balance between pro- and anti-inflammatory immune system messengers (cytokines), as well preventing white cells from crossing the blood–brain barrier and damaging myelin. It may also be due to interferon's effect on the cells that regulate the immune response (T-reg cells), and its suppression of those T cells that are primed to attack the body (auto-reactive T cells).

Side effects of interferons are common and can have a marked detrimental effect on quality of life. Most people develop flu-like symptoms on the day of injection, with fever, chills, muscle pain, nausea and perhaps vomiting and diarrhoea. The majority become more tolerant over time, but more serious side effects, such as liver and thyroid disease as well as depression, have also been documented. (These serious side effects necessitate regular blood monitoring.) Around one-third of patients develop hair loss, and injection site reactions are not uncommon. Pancreatitis is a rare but very serious side effect. Many people choose drugs with fewer side effects these days.

In 2018, long-term data demonstrated for the first time that those people taking interferons for ten years took four years longer to reach the point where they required the regular use of a cane (EDSS 6.0). Much of the benefit appeared to be derived from the first two years of treatment, which then gradually plateaued and was sustained.

Glatiramer acetate (Copaxone) was discovered in the 1960s by researchers trying to design a chemical capable of causing experimental autoimmune encephalitis (EAE, the animal equivalent of MS) in mice. What they found, however, was that glatiramer tricks the immune system into activating certain cells that once they cross into the brain will reduce the inflammation at the site of MS lesions. In a way treatment with glatiramer is similar to desensitisation injections taken by those with severe allergies. Glatiramer shifts the balance of the immune system from a pro-inflammatory Th1 response to an anti-inflammatory Th2 response, and also appears to have a neuro-protective role, protecting brain cells from damage. This effect tends to increase with long-term use of the drug. Like interferons, glatiramer reduces relapse rates by around one-third, and is usually administered as a daily or more potent second-daily self-injection.

Unlike the interferons, glatiramer generally causes very few side effects, with the exception of skin reactions, often due to incorrect injecting technique. Flushing, heart palpitations and shortness of breath are uncommonly experienced at the time of injection. Glatiramer does not suppress the immune system, and therefore does not leave the patient at increased risk of infection, unlike many of the other DMTs. It also requires no regular blood monitoring. Glatiramer is now thought to have a 'modest' effect on reduction of the risk of disability progression (16.5 per cent) compared to placebo, and importantly, its effectiveness does not appear to diminish over time.

First-generation injectables reduce relapse rates by around 30 per cent and modestly slow long-term disability progression; their use is limited by relatively minor but common and unpleasant side effects and more effective treatment options

The combination of side effects, modest efficacy and mode of delivery has meant the use of interferons and glatiramer has been largely superseded by the newer-generation DMTs, particularly the oral medications. They are, however, two of very few MS medications licensed for, and generally considered safe, in pregnancy and breastfeeding, with recent large-scale evidence showing no increase in pregnancy loss or foetal abnormalities compared to the general population.

Second-generation treatments
Oral therapies (teriflunomide, dimethyl fumarate, fingolimod, cladribine)

Teriflunomide (Aubagio) was approved for use in RRMS in 2012, taken as a once-daily tablet. It appears to reduce the MS immune response by stopping certain immune cells from multiplying. This results in lower numbers of both B cells and T cells, two types of white blood cells thought to be involved in the damage associated with MS. In studies, teriflunomide has been shown to reduce relapse rates by around 30 per cent compared to placebo.

Common side effects include nausea and vomiting, diarrhoea, pins and needles, hair loss, and respiratory and urinary tract infections. Raised liver enzyme levels are also associated, with rare cases of anaemia and low platelet levels. Regular blood monitoring is essential during treatment. It is also advised that people taking teriflunomide avoid alcohol and live vaccines.

Other than its relatively modest efficacy in MS, the significant factor limiting the use of teriflunomide is the risk of foetal abnormality, which persists for two years after stopping treatment. As most people with MS are women, and the majority are in the reproductive phase of their lives, this is often a key concern when choosing a DMT. Current advice is that women of child-bearing age should use an effective method of contraception during treatment. There is also evidence that teriflunomide is transmitted in semen, so men taking the medication are advised to use barrier contraceptive methods, continuing for two years after stopping treatment. In the event of pregnancy during treatment or the two-year wash-out period, a treatment can be given (cholestyramine or activated charcoal) to try to rapidly remove traces of the drug from the body.

Dimethyl fumarate (BG-12, Tecfidera) has been used safely for many years as a treatment for the autoimmune skin condition psoriasis. It was first approved in 2013 for use in RRMS and is taken as a twice-daily capsule. Dimethyl fumarate reduces the inflammation caused when the immune system attacks the myelin sheath, resulting in less damage to myelin. It also appears to protect nerve cells from damage caused by chemicals released during the immune attack.

Studies have demonstrated a relapse rate reduction of around 50 per cent compared to placebo, with a significant reduction in new lesions on MRI. There is evidence from one study (DEFINE trial) of slowing of disability progression at two years. Side effects include flushing, nausea and vomiting, diarrhoea, upper respiratory and urinary tract infections, and itching. Around

10 per cent of those taking the medication choose to stop due to its side effects. Dimethyl fumarate can cause a reduction in white blood cell count, as well as deranged liver and kidney function, so regular blood tests are performed during treatment.

A very rare side effect is progressive multifocal leukoencephalopathy (PML). To date there have been fewer than ten cases worldwide (a rate of 1/50,000), and this brain infection is more commonly associated with natalizumab (more information below). Nevertheless, it has the potential to cause severe disability or even death, but is generally only of concern if the lymphocyte count (a type of white blood cell) is very low for a prolonged period of time. Hence the need for regular blood monitoring. There is currently limited data available concerning dimethyl fumarate in pregnancy and breastfeeding, and while at this stage there are no specific concerns, both are advised to be avoided during treatment.

Fingolimod (Gilenya) was the first oral DMT approved for use in RRMS, and one of the most effective. It is a once-daily tablet and appears to work by trapping certain white blood cells (T cells) in the lymph nodes (akin to keeping soldiers locked in their barracks). These cells are involved in the immune response that damages myelin; trapping them in the lymph nodes results in fewer getting across the blood brain barrier to the brain and spinal cord. Interestingly, this process is not absolute, so the immune system can still mount a response against an outside invader if needed, and the patient is not overly immunosuppressed. In the original studies, fingolimod was shown to reduce relapse rates of 50–60 per cent compared to placebo, with significantly fewer new lesions on MRI and reduced rates of brain shrinkage (atrophy) in those taking the drug. The early evidence suggests that fingolimod may reduce the rate of disability progression.

Common side effects include increased risk of infections (colds and flu), cough, headache, back pain, diarrhoea and increased liver enzyme levels. Viral infections, particularly due to herpes viruses, are more common and more severe with fingolimod. It is therefore advised that people are vaccinated against varicella (the virus that causes chicken pox and shingles) before treatment, if not previously exposed.

Cases of basal cell carcinoma, a type of skin cancer, have been reported with fingolimod. This is a slow-growing skin cancer that almost never spreads, but can be disfiguring if not treated at an early stage. There have also been a very small number of reported cases of malignant melanoma, a much more serious skin cancer. Fingolimod may also cause the less common side effect of macular oedema, a swelling in the back of the eye that can affect vision.

The first dose of fingolimod is given in hospital with heart-rate monitoring. This is in case an abnormally slow heart rhythm develops, but this effect does not appear to occur with subsequent doses. People with pre-existing heart conditions are usually advised to avoid fingolimod, as it can reduce the force of contraction of the heart muscle.

A phenomenon particularly associated with fingolimod is that of 'rebound'. In around 10 per cent of people, when they stop taking the drug, either to switch to another DMT or stop completely, their MS 'rebounds' to the pre-treatment level. Rarely, their disease activity worsens, and there is research ongoing into which drug to switch to, and the length of time required between stopping fingolimod and starting the next.

Another key consideration when taking fingolimod is pregnancy. The risk of potentially toxic foetal side effects persist for two months after stopping the drug, and so reliable contraception should be used. Fingolimod has no effect on sperm count or motility and is present only in extremely low levels in semen, so there are no concerns regarding conception for men taking the medication. Breastfeeding is not recommended when taking fingolimod.

Cladribine (Mavenclad) is a chemotherapy agent approved for use in RRMS in 2017. It is a tablet, taken daily for up to five days, then again for up to five days the following month. This cycle is repeated after twelve months. To date, further courses of cladribine have not been required for those receiving two cycles of treatment, but this is currently being monitored on a more long-term basis.

Cladribine appears to work by targeting two types of white blood cell (B and T lymphocytes), destroying them temporarily. The immune system then rebuilds these cell populations, with the theory being that they will no longer target the myelin sheath. It doesn't seem to suppress the overall immune system significantly, so infections can still be fought, and nor does it appear to damage cells other than the white blood cells, so there are fewer side effects.

Cladribine was put forward for approval in 2010, but withdrawn due to initial concerns over increased numbers of cancers in the treatment group. It is now felt that cladribine does not increase an individual's risk of cancer. In clinical trials there was a reduction in relapse rate of 58 per cent compared to placebo. Later analyses found that the rate of brain volume loss was reduced and the number of participants with no evidence of disease activity (NEDA) was also increased in those taking cladribine. Early evidence suggests that cladribine slows disability accumulation by around 30 per cent.

Potential side effects include decreased white blood cell count, more frequent herpes virus infections (including shingles) and hair loss. Blood tests are routinely performed three and seven months after treatment. Tests are also carried out before receiving cladribine to exclude tuberculosis, HIV and hepatitis.

Both men and women are advised to avoid pregnancy and use reliable contraception for six months after their last dose of cladribine, given the potential risk of foetal abnormalities.

The oral DMTs reduce relapses by around 30–60 per cent, and are often used as a first-line treatment in RRMS

Infusions (natalizumab, alemtuzumab, ocrelizumab)

The infusion-based medications currently form the 'highest level' of routine DMT treatment, and are associated with the greatest effect in terms of reducing disease activity. They also come with the most significant risks and side-effect profile. They are administered as an intravenous preparation, some on a regular basis ranging from once a month to every six months, while others are given as a single course, split over twelve months.

Natalizumab (Tysabri) is an intravenous infusion given every four weeks and is licensed for RRMS. It reduces relapse rates by 70 per cent compared to placebo and has been shown to slow disability progression. It works by binding to a receptor on immune cells (alpha 4 integrin) and prevents them from getting into the brain and spinal cord to damage myelin.

Common side effects include dizziness, inflammation of the nose and throat, nausea, vomiting, skin rash, shivering and an increased chance of infection. Natalizumab may affect liver function but this generally recovers when treatment is stopped. The most significant consideration when starting treatment with natalizumab, however, is that it can increase the risk of the brain infection PML. This can lead to severe disability or even death in up to 25 per cent of those affected. PML is caused by a mutation of the JC virus, a common infection completely unrelated to MS. Between 50 and 70 per cent of the general population have been exposed to the JC virus, and it is normally kept completely under control by the immune system, causing no symptoms.

But if the immune system is weakened and the body is less able to fight infection, which may occur with natalizumab, the JC virus can become active and cause inflammation and damage to the brain. A blood test can detect the presence of the JC virus and give an indication of the level of risk that one might develop PML (e.g. 1 in 1000 chance). Other factors that increase the risk of PML include previous treatment with an immunosuppressant drug and the length of time taking natalizumab (the risk increases after two years or more of treatment). Your neurologist or MS nurse should discuss the implications of the blood test and how it may influence a decision for or against treatment. If you are negative for the JC virus, the risk of PML is extremely low (around 1 in 10,000), but you can encounter the JC virus at any time, so this should be checked every six months.

When starting natalizumab, all patients should be made aware of the early signs and symptoms of PML. These can be similar to an MS relapse, so it is important to report any new or worsening symptoms. If PML is suspected at any point, the drug will be discontinued immediately. New evidence is emerging that 'extended interval dosing'—that is, increasing the time between each treatment from four weeks to between five and eight weeks—effectively reduces the risk of PML while maintaining protection against MS disease activity. In those with a higher body mass index (BMI), the shorter interval appears to be safer and different health authorities will apply different criteria in making a decision on dosing intervals.

If one has to stop natalizumab, for example due to side effects or increasing risk of PML, there is a chance that, as with fingolimod, MS can rebound and become more active than before starting natalizumab. At least 10 per cent of patients stopping natalizumab may develop this rebound phenomenon, usually between twelve and sixteen weeks after the last dose of natalizumab. The key then is to give the next DMT at the right time—too soon and the immune system will be severely compromised, too late and MS activity may significantly increase. There is currently research underway to establish which of the other DMTs may be able to control this increased MS activity, but it appears that the risk of rebound is highest when only using natalizumab for a few cycles and then stopping, rather than using it longer term. At present, many neurologists will switch patients to ocrelizumab as a next step.

Natalizumab is generally considered safe in pregnancy, and for many people with MS the risk associated with stopping suddenly outweighs any risk to the foetus. There are no specific associated birth defects or pregnancy complications, and the medication is often continued until 34 weeks of pregnancy to minimise the risk of rebound disease activity. There is also a very low level of absorption in breastmilk, and a consensus group of neurologists has considered it safe to breastfeed while taking natalizumab.

Alemtuzumab (Lemtrada) has been licensed for use in RRMS since 2014. It is given as an intravenous infusion over five days, then twelve months later as a second course over three days. It was initially stated that no further treatment was necessary, but more recent follow-up data has shown that up to 50 per cent of patients require a third or fourth dose. Alemtuzumab reduces relapse rates by around 70 per cent compared to placebo, with evidence for slowing of disability progression, and in some cases even an improvement of disability levels.

It is sometimes thought of as a 'mini stem-cell transplant' because alemtuzumab binds to both B and T cells and permanently destroys them. It is believed that new B and T cells are manufactured in the bone marrow that the immune system repopulates without knowledge that it was previously primed to attack myelin. For this reason alemtuzumab is classed as an immune reconstitution therapy (IRT), and once administered causes permanent immune system changes.

While highly effective as a treatment for MS, alemtuzumab has a very significant side-effect profile. It is known that between one-fifth and up to one-half of patients will develop secondary autoimmunity as a result of treatment (the 'new' immune system that grows back attacks another part of the body). The most common is an autoimmune thyroid condition that can be lifelong and require medical treatment in its own right. Around 1–3 per cent of patients develop a bleeding disorder, idiopathic thrombocytopaenic purpura, where the immune system attacks platelets in the blood stream. This is potentially serious but usually treatable. Autoimmune kidney disease has also been reported. Monthly blood monitoring is required for four years following the last dose of alemtuzumab to detect these autoimmune adverse events.

Less serious but more common side effects include nausea, headaches, rash, hives, fever, itching, insomnia and fatigue. Additional medications are given at the time of the infusion to minimise these. Certain infections involving the lungs, sinuses and urinary tract and related to the herpes virus are more common following alemtuzumab treatment. Antiviral treatment is given for at least a month following a treatment cycle to reduce this risk.

In 2019, new concerns emerged regarding alemtuzumab and previously unknown side effects involving the liver, heart, blood vessels and immune system. While rare, these can be very serious, and as a result the use of the drug has been restricted in many countries to those people with more aggressive forms of RRMS, with rapidly evolving symptoms or worsening disease activity despite taking at least one DMT.

Before starting treatment, certain vaccinations may be required, and you will be advised on necessary precautions in the months following treatment to reduce the risk of infection as a result of immunosuppression while the immune system repopulates. As the situation is rapidly evolving, check with your neurologist about the latest advice with regard to COVID vaccination. Women are advised to avoid pregnancy for at least four months after a treatment course, and should not receive a course while breastfeeding.

Ocrelizumab (Ocrevus), approved in 2018, is the first DMT licensed to treat primary progressive MS (PPMS) and can also be used in RRMS. While its availability for PPMS is by no means universal at present, and the restrictive eligibility criteria in certain jurisdictions are a source of much frustration for the MS community, nonetheless it is still a hugely significant step on the road towards meaningful treatments for people living with progressive forms of MS.

Ocrelizumab acts by targeting a marker (CD20) on the B cell, thought to be involved in the abnormal immune response that attacks the myelin coating of nerve cells. In both forms of the disease, it is given as an intravenous infusion every six months, with the first dose split over two weeks.

In clinical trials for PPMS, the group of people taking ocrelizumab reduced their chance of worsening disability after twelve weeks by one-quarter (24 per cent), compared to those taking a placebo. While this may not sound like a huge difference, it is the first medication ever to show a statistically significant improvement in outcomes in PPMS. After two years of treatment, walking speed had slowed less than in the placebo group, and there were also fewer brain lesions and brain shrinkage (atrophy) in the treatment group. It will be extremely interesting to see how these improvements will be borne out over the long term, and what it means for people living with PPMS.

When used for treating RRMS, ocrelizumab reduced the number of relapses by 50 per cent compared to interferon-beta, reduced disability progression sustained for three and six months, and significantly reduced the number of lesions seen on MRI scans compared to interferon. The rate of brain volume loss was reduced, and there were more people with no evidence of disease activity (NEDA) in the ocrelizumab treatment groups.

It is generally very well tolerated, with no unexpected side effects reported in the phase III trials. That said, it is not without risks, and these typically include infusion site reactions, chest infections, cold sores and shingles (due to herpes virus infections). Opportunistic infections such as those caused by bacteria and viruses normally kept under control by the immune system are also more common. There is a potentially increased risk of some cancers, but this as yet not confirmed and is being closely monitored. This risk is not unique to ocrelizumab, but a possible side effect of many drugs that alter the immune system.

The infusion-based DMTs are highly effective at reducing disease activity, and appear to significantly reduce disability accumulation if given early in the disease course. However, they have significant, sometimes severe side effects

A recent large-scale review compared ocrelizumab with the other available DMTs and found that it fared very favourably in terms of side effects and safety profile. It was also at least as effective, if not more so, than all the other medications tested. Ocrelizumab is in fact a slightly altered version of the older drug rituximab (Rituxan), a treatment for lymphomas and leukaemias. This has been used in the treatment of MS for some years in countries such as Sweden, where a large registry of patients has shown an excellent safety record and efficacy in the real-world setting.

Treatments for progressive MS (siponimod, ofatumumab, ocrelizumab)

As previously mentioned, ocrelizumab (Ocrevus) is now licensed in many countries as a treatment for both RRMS and PPMS. Hopefully, over the coming months and years it will become more widely available for use in PPMS, as more long-term evidence demonstrates its sustained effects and benefits, thereby confirming its cost-effectiveness.

There are currently two other DMTs that are into the final stages of receiving licensing approval, and many more at earlier stages of research and development.

Siponimod (Mayzent) is a once-daily tablet, now licensed for the treatment of secondary progressive MS (SPMS) in the United States and Europe. Similar to ocrelizumab, it is currently only available to specific patients, usually those with 'active' SPMS, meaning that there is evidence of disease activity on MRI, or that they still experience relapses. It comes from the same family as fingolimod (both are S1P receptor modulators). Siponimod blocks the release of white blood cells from the lymph nodes, thereby reducing the autoimmune attack in the brain and spinal cord, with a similar side effect profile to its older relative.

In clinical trials (e.g. EXPAND), siponimod was found to reduce the risk of confirmed disability progression by 31 per cent at three months, and by 37 per cent at six months, compared to placebo. There were also significant favourable differences in other measures of MS disease activity, including a reduction in relapse rate and less disease activity and brain volume loss (atrophy) on MRI. It was also found to provide clinically significant benefits in cognitive processing speeds, and reduced the chance of cognitive decline over the five-year follow-up period.

Ofatumumab (Kesimpta) is now licensed in the United States for the treatment of RRMS and active SPMS and going through approval processes in other countries. Previously administered as a high-dose infusion in certain types of leukaemia, in MS it has the advantage of being given by self-injection under the skin once a month. Ofatumumab acts in a similar way to ocrelizumab (anti-CD20 monoclonal antibody), preventing B lymphocytes from attacking the brain and spinal cord, but can be given at home, rather than every six months in a hospital or clinic.

In recent studies (ASCLEPIOS I and II), ofatumumab was compared with the oral treatment teriflunomide (Aubagio) in people with RRMS and active SPMS over a follow-up period of two and a half years. Ofatumumab led to a 97.5 per cent relative reduction in the number of MRI lesions in ASCLEPIOS I, and 93.8 per cent in ASCLEPIOS II, relative to teriflunomide. In terms of disability progression, the risk was reduced by 34.4 per cent at three months, and 32.5 per cent at six months with ofatumumab, compared with teriflunomide.

Common side effects include upper respiratory tract infections, injection-related reactions such as fever, headache, muscle pain, chills and fatigue, and local injection site reactions such as redness, pain, itching and swelling. There were no significant differences between the two groups with regard to the rate of infections or cancers.

Future research developments

The recent increase in progressive MS research and treatments is very welcome. The global MS research community has now recognised the urgent need for a better understanding of the processes that underpin MS disease progression, which in turn will reveal further potential treatment targets. The International Progressive MS Alliance now includes eighteen global MS charities, with the overall goal of speeding up treatment development, and there are ambitious targets to stop disease progression and even reverse disability. In the United Kingdom the MS Society has committed to having treatments for all forms of MS by 2025.

Broadly speaking, there are three key areas that scientists are currently investigating in their efforts to gain a better understanding of MS, and to develop safer and more effective treatments.

Preventing damage by the immune system

If it were possible to stop the immune system from mistakenly attacking myelin, then relapses wouldn't occur and disability would not progress. At present, however, scientists do not fully understand why the immune system malfunctions in MS. Until that puzzle is unlocked, the DMTs generally operate by rather crude mechanisms, trying to control the immune attack by the processes of immunosuppression or immunomodulation. While they can trap white blood cells in lymph nodes, or destroy certain cell types, this in turn affects other parts of the exquisitely complex immune system, leaving the patient with side effects or at risk of complications such as infections, PML or even cancers.

There are many areas being explored in this regard. One example is the role of vitamin D in the normal functioning of the immune system (see Chapter 4 by Dr Conor Kerley for more detail), and whether increasing levels in someone with MS alters the disease activity.

Another example is haematopoietic stem cell transplantation (HSCT). An extremely aggressive treatment, very similar to that used in a bone marrow transplant, the patient's own stem cells are collected and stored, before a chemotherapy treatment is given that completely wipes out their immune system. The original stem cells are then reinfused. The theory is that the newly formed system has been 'rebooted', with no memory of MS, and therefore will not attack myelin.

Early evidence suggests that it can halt the disease in the short to medium term, and may reverse disability in some people, generally those who have early and inflammatory forms of the condition with relatively low levels of disease progression, but more research is needed before it can be considered a mainstream treatment.

The regimen involved is very physically and emotionally demanding, with lengthy periods of complete isolation as the immune system reconstitutes (often in hospital), on average a 6–12-month recovery time frame after discharge, and at present up to 1 per cent chance of dying from the procedure due to infection and bleeding disorders. One must also be very wary of the 'health tourism' that often comes with HSCT, where clinics in certain countries offer potentially unproven or less well-regulated treatments for often substantial sums of money.

Promoting myelin repair (remyelination)

This is sometimes seen as the 'holy grail' of MS research. If you could rebuild or repair damaged myelin, then MS symptoms and disability could be significantly reduced or even reversed. Finding treatments that repair myelin could also work alongside drugs that aim to prevent an immune attack. When myelin is attacked, special cells within the brain and spinal cord, called oligodendrocytes, are signalled to migrate to the site of damage and repair the injury. The newly repaired myelin can then function again, and this often leads to a reduction or resolution of neurological symptoms. Early in the course of MS, this process works relatively well, but over time it becomes less effective, so that recovery is less complete from each relapse, and disability can progress. If treatments can be found to keep the oligodendrocytes and their stem cell precursors (OPCs) active, then there is real potential for useful treatments in both relapsing and progressive forms of MS.

Several drugs already in use for other conditions have shown early promise in this regard, and are now in clinical trials. An over-the-counter antihistamine, clemastine (not available in Australia), has been found to increase nerve transmission speed in a nerve in the eye (optic nerve) of people with MS and is again being studied to establish whether taking it can improve MS symptoms and disability.

Low-dose naltrexone (LDN) is another example, already used by many people with MS, owing to its low cost, minimal side effects and excellent safety record. It was designed to treat opiate overdoses (morphine and heroin), but when given in a much lower dose it appears to prevent oligodendrocyte cell death. There are small studies and anecdotal reports suggesting that it reduces relapses and can even reverse symptoms with long-term use. Unfortunately, large-scale studies are unlikely to occur, as it is a generic drug and drug companies are unwilling to invest in non-patentable drugs.

Protecting nerves from damage (neuroprotection)

Protecting nerves from damage is a key area in slowing disease progression and, importantly, these therapies could be effective regardless of MS subtype. Once the myelin sheath is injured, the underlying nerve fibre is vulnerable to damage and death from the myelin debris and other toxic substances. Once the nerve fibre dies (axonal loss) it cannot be replaced and signals can no longer be transmitted, which in turn can lead to permanent disability.

Nerve cell death is a normal part of ageing, but happens much faster in people with MS. It can be seen on MRI scans as brain shrinkage (atrophy), and is increasingly being monitored in trials for new DMTs and other treatments as a marker of MS disease activity.

One such drug is simvastatin, currently being studied in the MS-STAT 2 trial in the United Kingdom. Statins are very commonly prescribed to reduce blood cholesterol levels. In MS, early research showed that simvastatin reduced inflammation and protected nerves from damage, as well as slowing brain atrophy rates by 43 per cent. The current trial aims to establish whether this can slow, stop or improve disability progression in people with SPMS.

Mastinib is a twice-daily tablet that has been specifically designed to treat primary and secondary progressive MS, and is in the final stages of clinical trials. Results have shown that those with PPMS and non-active SPMS (not experiencing relapses) had a slower rate of disability progression than those taking placebo, while being safe and well tolerated. This is extremely promising, given the current lack of treatments available for progressive MS.

Another example is ibudilast, an oral asthma drug commonly used in Japan and Korea. Early studies in PPMS (e.g. SPRINT-MS) have shown that it slowed brain volume loss by 48 per cent compared to placebo over two years. MRI studies also revealed that ibudilast had a protective role against myelin and nerve damage. Further trials are now being designed to determine its effects on disability and cognition, as well as for those with SPMS.

Points to consider if starting a DMT

For some people living with MS, using a DMT is a key component of their recovery and in maintaining their health. For others, a DMT may not be available to them at all due to local healthcare resources, cost or their own particular type of MS. There will also be many people who simply feel that using a DMT is not the right decision for them. Regardless of MS type, healthcare provider or DMT use, the preventive medicine lifestyle changes discussed in this book should form a key part of your own journey towards lifelong good health and living well with MS.

Choosing to use a DMT is not a decision that should be rushed. This is a drug that you will potentially take for many years, possibly the rest of your life. While many neurologists now believe in starting aggressive treatment as soon as possible after diagnosis, this is a lifelong, chronic condition and it is extremely important to make a decision that feels right for you, and that you can live with.

First of all, it is important to get a sense from your medical team about how active the MS is, and be guided by them as to which medications are available and appropriate for you, and which type (oral, infusion, injectable) they advise. Then do your own research, using reputable sources such as local MS charity websites and information leaflets.

As part of the decision-making process, if you do decide to take one of the DMTs, it may be helpful to consider the following points, and perhaps even draw up a list of the pros and cons of each individual drug.

When should I start?
Do I have a particularly aggressive form of MS and need to get things under control as quickly as possible, or can I afford to wait until I have another MRI scan or clinic review, while changing my lifestyle?

Which one should I take?
Based on my circumstances, which DMTs are available and which ones is my doctor advising?

What benefits can I expect?

How long will it take for the drug to start working, and how effective is it likely to be in reducing the number and/or severity of relapses? Is it likely to help slow down disability progression?

What are the risks and potential side effects?

Is taking a particular drug going to help me feel better day to day, without noticeable effects, or are there potentially unpleasant, debilitating or even dangerous side effects?

How will it fit into my lifestyle?

Does the medication need to be kept in a refrigerator? Can I take it on a plane if I need to travel? Do I need to remember to eat before taking it? Will I need to remember to take it twice daily? Do I have to learn how to inject myself and dispose of needles? Will I have to make sure I can get to the hospital every month for an infusion?

What monitoring will I need?

How often will I need to have blood tests performed, if at all, and will I need regular MRI scans—every six months; twelve months?

What about starting a family?

Can I get pregnant while taking this medication? Would there be any risks to the baby if I got pregnant accidentally? How long would I have to wait before trying to conceive after treatment? Can I breastfeed?

Overall, there have been great advances in pharmaceutical treatment for MS, but the drugs remain only modestly effective and many have significant side effects that may not be acceptable to many people with MS. Take time and make a carefully weighted decision about whether to take a DMT and, if so, which one. In the meantime, get started immediately with lifestyle changes.

Ground covered

The advances in medical treatments for MS have been rapid over the past twenty years. There are ever-increasing options for RRMS and progressive forms of the condition, although widespread availability remains an issue.

Evidence is increasingly demonstrating that the use of relatively high-efficacy DMTs early in the disease course offers the best chances of reduced disability progression over time. However, the more effective a DMT, generally the greater the risks and side-effect profile, and this is something to consider.

The next 5–10 years will almost certainly yield a large number of new and more effective treatment options, including those for progressive forms of MS. There is every reason to believe that scientists will also develop treatments that can slow, stop or even reverse disability progression. But even if a 'cure' is discovered, the role of lifestyle modification will remain just as important in maintaining lifelong good health, and in living well with MS.

My Story:
Dr Catriona Tate PhD

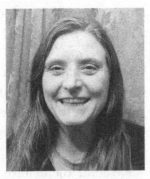

We're all on the same journey, but everybody has a different path. MS affects each of us very differently, in terms of symptoms and progression. The OMS Program provides a map for a route to better health. Most guidelines are the same for everyone; medication is rather different. Each individual needs to consider the potential risks and benefits of specific treatments (which vary a lot) in conjunction with their medical team. It can be a tough choice, but it isn't a 'forever decision'. Some people (like George Jelinek) take medication then stop when they feel their condition is under control (or change treatment to improve outcomes). Some people decide to wait and see whether they need medication. I took Tysabri for five years, stopped for two years during pregnancy and breastfeeding (this was the medical advice although now it's possible to continue this treatment through pregnancy), then restarted. Over time I've reduced the frequency of doses.

MS for me started halfway through my PhD. I lost all feeling in my hands, starting at the tips of my right fingers, and gradually spreading up both arms, then into my legs. A spate of nosebleeds led to an MRI scan to rule out MS or an aggressive brain tumour. As soon as I heard I had MS, it made sense. I remembered an incident six years earlier when I lost feeling in my hands but was dismissed as hysterical, before the symptoms vanished as mysteriously as they arrived (I assumed it was a trapped nerve).

Then they came back with a vengeance. Diagnosis was a relief. I was sad but thought, this time they listened, and it's not brain cancer, and I have something to research. Alongside other books and articles, I read *Taking Control of Multiple Sclerosis* (2nd ed, 2005) by George Jelinek. I liked George's focus on ways to help himself, and that he had cited all of his (hundreds of) sources. I read some of the same original research and agreed with his conclusions. I thought, 'I have to try this!'

My symptoms were worsening rapidly, in a terrifying downward spiral. Every few weeks there was a new blow. I couldn't tell what positions my limbs were in without looking. I lost feeling in patches of skin on my torso. My limbs would jerk and flail uncontrollably. I slurred my speech. I dropped or broke things (I couldn't tell how hard I was holding anything). I couldn't write my name, or dress myself unaided. This all happened within four months and was getting worse. I changed my diet, I exercised, but I needed something more rapid. Steroids brought me some breathing space, then I started Tysabri.

Eleven years later, I have recovered more than I would have dreamed was possible. I danced with my husband at our wedding, finished my PhD, continued working full-time, had a child. I can walk, even run. Pilates helped greatly. I can write. I have no regrets about following the OMS Program or starting on Tysabri. I think they gave my body the chance to recover, and to learn how to send nerve signals along different pathways. One thing I am grateful for is that the Program gave me choices . . . and I used them.

8

Progressive MS

Dr Philip Startin

> If I had discovered OMS when I was first diagnosed with MS, my journey with MS would surely have been a whole lot easier; however, even with secondary progressive MS my quality of life has improved after reading the book and subscribing to the OMS website.
>
> *Jayne McClure, Sydney, Australia, OMSer*

Of the different forms of MS, progressive multiple sclerosis (PMS) is the least common at onset, generally occurs slightly later in life, and affects women and men in equal numbers. It is also the least understood, both in terms of underlying mechanisms and outcomes. It is typically portrayed very negatively, often as the 'worst' type of MS. PMS results in the gradual loss of physical and cognitive function: for primary progressive MS (PPMS) from onset of the condition and for secondary progressive MS (SPMS) following a series of relapses. However, the rate of loss is hugely variable from person to person, and functional loss typically happens slowly over decades.

Perhaps its uncertain course and unrelenting nature is why PMS is sometimes considered to be the most challenging form of MS. So looking after one's physical and mental health becomes even more important, arguably even more so than for the relapsing form. Even with PMS there are things that can be done to affect the trajectory of the condition, slow progression, even recover some lost function, and live well.

About progressive MS

When MS was originally categorised into different clinical subtypes, two were adopted: progressive MS (PMS) and relapsing remitting MS (RRMS). It was in 1996 that PMS was subdivided into PPMS and SPMS, and it is only the onset of these two subtypes that differs, with the onset of SPMS following from RRMS. This chapter deals with PMS in general.

The majority of MS research has focused on the more common relapsing form, and consequently this form is much better understood and there are far more disease-modifying therapies (DMTs) available for it. Until recently, PMS had few DMTs available and seemed almost to be secondary in importance and consideration to RRMS. But the progressive form of the condition has recently become an increased focus of research. As the understanding of PMS increases, new treatments and interventions are being identified, and neurologists are now even challenging the fundamental understanding of what MS actually is.

So how is PMS different?

The course of MS is highly variable, and symptoms and rate of progression can vary hugely from person to person. As indicated above, a number of MS subtypes have traditionally been used to categorise the condition within people with *broadly* similar symptoms: PPMS, SPMS and RRMS.

The features of RRMS were described by Dr Brandon Beaber in Chapter 1, 'Understanding multiple sclerosis'. This form of MS is driven by the classic MS cycle of inflammatory damage and consequential demyelination, the damage to or loss of the white 'fatty' myelin sheath that protects the axons, the 'wires' inside the central nervous system (CNS) that form the connections between neurons. It is the myelin-coated axons that form the 'white matter' that one can see in the brain, the white actually being the myelin. And the grey matter seen in the brain is mainly composed of the (grey-coloured) nerve cell bodies.

It is this inflammatory-driven demyelination that leads to the clinical symptoms of RRMS, and subsequent remyelination (myelin repair) that provides some of the partial or complete recovery. For some, after living with RRMS for a number of years, this condition becomes progressive and symptoms cause subsequent progressive deterioration, the subtype of MS defined as SPMS.

Although MRI scans are generally not a pleasant experience (being trapped in a confined, noisy, metal tube for 30 minutes or longer), MRI scanners provide an effective means of investigating the 'scars' (or sclerosis) left in the white matter of the brain as a consequence of the inflammation, and these multiple 'scars' on the white matter in the brain are why MS has traditionally been thought of as a white matter disease of the central nervous system. Having a better understanding of the inflammatory mechanisms that underlie RRMS as well as having good tools to diagnose and track this form of the condition has facilitated the development of a number of DMTs for RRMS.

However, more recently it has been reported that 'scars' detected on the MRI scans do not closely correspond with loss of physical and cognitive function in people with RRMS. It is now suggested that most overall disability accumulation in RRMS is due to an underlying progressive disease course, and that relapses and the white matter 'scars' are only weakly correlated with accumulated loss of function.

MS is a complex neurological condition that is still not well understood, and PMS particularly so; but this is changing and major insights into PMS are being made

The trajectory of PMS is different. Here disease progression and loss of function are relentless from the onset, although the pace of progression is hugely variable between individuals. In PMS it is neurodegeneration and loss of the grey matter (atrophy) in the CNS that is occurring, and it is this grey matter loss that leads to increasing physical and cognitive disability. It is still unclear how, or even whether, this atrophy of the CNS is linked to the inflammatory processes seen in RRMS.

The types of MRI scans used to investigate white matter damage caused by RRMS are not so helpful in determining the loss of grey matter caused in PMS. Neurologists are still trying to determine the mechanisms that drive this degeneration of the grey matter and to find a way to both accurately diagnose PMS and to measure progression. This partly explains why there are currently so few DMTs for those of us with PMS.

Is MS an inflammatory or a degenerative condition? Or both?

Most of the diagrams about MS seen on MS-related websites show the inflammation of the myelin sheath around the nerves and the consequential demyelination. But what about loss of the nerve cells (neurons) themselves—the degeneration of the grey matter? And are these two processes linked?

MS has been traditionally thought of as an initially inflammatory demyelinating condition, presenting as RRMS, which then drives the neurodegenerative process, as seen in PPMS and SPMS (the two subtypes of PMS). Some neurologists now suggest that perhaps MS is actually a degenerative condition, with inflammation occurring as a secondary response. Research has found that degeneration is also present in RRMS, so early treatment and looking after brain health are important for all with MS, not just those with PMS, and that the majority of disease accumulation in RRMS is actually caused by degeneration and not as a result of inflammation. Furthermore, inflammation can be present in PMS in addition to the more dominant mechanism of degeneration, so relapses can still occur even with the progressive forms of MS.

Some neurologists are now suggesting that we should think of MS as a continuum, or a spectrum, with more inflammation and demyelination in the RRMS cases and more degeneration in PMS, so these two 'dimensions' would position us each uniquely on the MS spectrum, better reflecting the very individual nature of the condition. Figure 8.1 provides an illustration of this.

MS professionals are increasingly describing the condition as 'active' or not, and whether there has been 'progression' or

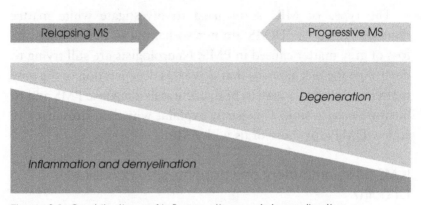

Figure 8.1: Contributions of inflammation and demyelination compared with degeneration in relapsing remitting vs progressive MS types. Source: Progressive Multiple Sclerosis by D. Ontaneda & R.J. Fox, in *Current Opinion in Neurology*, 2015.

Does MS start with inflammation or degeneration? Both are probably present, in varying degrees, at all stages and all forms of the condition

not. 'Activity' refers to relapses and the appearance of new damage to the white matter associated with inflammation and demyelination. 'Progression' refers to loss of physical (and cognitive) function caused by degeneration and loss of grey matter. So perhaps over the next few years the labels of RRMS, SPMS and PPMS will disappear and be replaced with terms that more closely reflect the more complete understanding of MS that MS professionals are developing.

Living with a 'new normal'

Regardless of the mechanism, PMS very typically results in a gradual loss of physical and cognitive functions. The hard and difficult truth is that it is highly likely that if you have PMS then you will lose some function over time. *But what is not certain is the rate of change, and those of us with PMS are not often told that there are things we can do to alter the trajectory of the change.*

A diagnosis of PMS is often portrayed as the 'worst-case scenario' of anyone who is diagnosed with MS, although the rate of change of function and type of change vary hugely between individuals. As the case study of Dave Jackman at the end of this chapter shows, some do live with PMS for decades and show very slow, gradual, or even no discernible loss of function. Statistically, the majority of those with PMS show more loss of function, but progression is typically slow, as in my case. Unfortunately, however, a small number do lose function a lot faster.

It is likely that if you have PMS, what is 'normal' for you will change over months and years. But this is unlikely to be linear, both in terms of how quickly things change and what changes. So obviously coming to terms with this progressive and uncertain condition can be particularly difficult. And often the secondary impact of these changes is what will affect day-to-day lives—the ability to work and to enjoy personal and professional relationships. So emotional resilience and mental strength become particularly important.

Physical and cognitive changes might be slow, and sometimes show improvement, but there might be an awareness of a gradual loss of function over years. And many of us with PMS might experience a gradual loss of function accompanied by a cycle of loss and improvement in function on a periodic basis.

People with PMS often find that infections and other illnesses can be very debilitating. Unfortunately infections are actually more frequent in people with MS, and even more so in those with the progressive form of the condition. Urinary tract infections (UTIs) seem an especially common problem, because of frequently occurring bladder disturbance, and respiratory infections are also frustratingly frequent.

Although progression can be very slow, it is likely that if you have MS you will have to live with a 'new normal'; coming to terms with this can be difficult, particularly if your 'normal' is ever changing

The presence of an infection can have a huge impact on physical function and require longer periods of recovery than in the general population. But full function is typically restored after an infection, although it can feel frightening at the time. Even a simple cold can have a significant, although temporary, impact on MS symptoms. So looking after physical and mental health and keeping as well as possible are important from many different perspectives and can make a real difference.

Alter the trajectory

Although the reality is that being diagnosed with PMS usually means a gradual loss in physical and cognitive function over time, *it is possible to make lifestyle changes and alter the trajectory of the progression, and it is possible to even recover some lost function—both cognitive and physical.*

When Professor George Jelinek developed his OMS approach over twenty years ago, it was regarded as revolutionary. However, now, virtually wherever you are in the world and regardless of whether you have PMS or RRMS, your neurologist or MS professional will probably recommend some combination of a healthy diet, adequate vitamin D, exercise, and looking after your mental health. So OMS is thankfully becoming mainstream!

All the steps recommended in the OMS Program can help slow neurodegeneration and protect neurological function, as well as reduce inflammation. It's probably even more important to 'do whatever it takes' when living with the progressive form of the condition as slowing neurodegeneration and protecting the brain, and thereby minimising the gradual loss of mental and physical function, are critical. As pointed out earlier in this chapter, since demyelination and relapses may be present in the progressive subtype, minimising inflammation is still important.

The body's ability to recover lost function is amazing, and the 'plastic' nature of the brain and CNS is truly phenomenal. So even with PMS it is possible to recover some lost function. I have certainly experienced this personally, as have many others with PMS.

It does require effort and time. Trying to teach the mind and body new skills and literally rewire parts of our brain requires both lots of practice and high-quality practice. Paying such particular attention to 'form' when practising can be exhausting—not just physically tiring but also neurologically tiring as we're teaching the brain new ways to work and (re)learning new skills. ('Form' means that when exercising to retain or restore function, the brain needs to relearn the 'right' movement.)

Altering the trajectory of PMS requires a holistic effort, as exemplified by the OMS Program. We need to make sure that we eat well and eat food that does not promote degeneration and inflammation. Given the links between mind and body, as discussed extensively in Chapter 6 of this book, we need to look after our mind and learn how better to respond skilfully to the changes that will arise.

By rigorously following the OMS Program, I have personally seen some functional recovery as well as slowing overall progression. This has been observed in many others with PMS who have made lifestyle changes that include exercising more, eating better and looking after their mental health.

But we are all unique and how the condition progresses over time is individual for us all. Some will recover more function than others, and some will change the trajectory of the condition more than others *independent* of the amount of effort and determination put in. Perhaps this is because of the extent of 'brain reserve' we have remaining, both cognitive and neurological. But regardless of where we start from, all of us with PMS can make a positive difference to the trajectory of this condition.

> *It is possible to alter the trajectory of MS progression, both to slow progression and even recover some lost function*

Lifestyle modifications for PMS

Exercise

Unlike a couple of decades ago when people with MS were typically discouraged from exercising, exercise is now widely accepted as being particularly important to people with MS. For those with PMS the importance of exercise is even greater, and is critical to maintaining and even restoring function. The expression 'use it or lose it' is very pertinent for those with PMS.

Exercise helps in a number of different ways. Exercising preserves and develops muscular strength and endurance. It is well documented that exercise improves the immune response, protecting against viruses and infections, and can actually reduce neurodegeneration. And because of the amazing capability of the brain to develop new neural pathways throughout life, some lost function can actually be recovered. Recent research has begun to highlight the importance of comorbidities, the diseases that are commonly present alongside MS, and how these comorbidities can worsen the progression of MS. These include heart disease as well as other autoimmune conditions, which can also be positively affected by exercise.

Chapter 5 of this book by Dr Stuart White explores exercise in general for people with MS, and how to adopt a new exercise program and choose the right program, but are there any particular considerations for those with PMS?

As with the general population, strength and cardiovascular exercises are helpful and should be part of the exercise plan of anyone with PMS. These types of exercises are good for physical health, mental wellbeing and in preserving physical function. And if a particular part or side of the body seems to be having difficulty there are exercises that can address certain areas.

There are also exercises more focused on preserving and recovering function (e.g. foot drop or improving gait), and these might be suggested by a neurological physiotherapist. These functional exercises are important and also should be part of the exercise program, particularly if you have weakening physical function. And this includes core exercises too, another typical area of weakness for people with PMS.

But when performing all exercises, remember that form is key, so try and get support and guidance in how to perform the exercise 'correctly'. It is very common when exercising to hit a 'neurological edge', so becoming cognitively tired before becoming physically tired, which may affect form, so it's important to respect this too.

Another common symptom of PMS is a loss of proprioception—of knowing the position and movement of the body. This can cause clumsiness, poor balance and difficulty controlling posture. Loss of proprioception makes it more difficult to exercise correctly and maintain the right form. As mentioned before, form is key but it can be hard to exercise correctly: firstly, because of hitting the neurological edge and, secondly, because of loss of proprioception. So it's important to exercise to develop proprioception and also be mindful of not becoming too tired. Specific exercises and movement can help the body relearn how to control itself better and eliminate some of these issues.

What can also help are general outdoor physical activities, and there are lots of adaptive sports that can be tried—rowing, skiing, horse riding, to name a few. The available adaptations are amazing and almost anyone with any degree of loss of physical function can find a sport or exercise they can participate in. Plus, doing a sport outdoors can really be fun, help switch on production of endorphins and serotonin, and just make you feel better and more connected.

Like most people who exercise you are likely to have goals: how far or fast are you going to walk, how long can you stand for, how many pullups are you going to be able to do by the end of the year? With PMS it is important to have clear goals but you may need to learn how to hold these firmly and at the same time lightly, and to be more accepting if sometimes goals are not achieved without letting this affect commitment and motivation. It does take time to relearn new skills and rewire the brain and there may be

Exercise slows neurodegeneration and is important in maintaining physical function; it can help preserve strength and mobility, improve emotional wellbeing and actually recover some lost function

periods when exercising is more difficult. Also remember to celebrate the smaller achievements too—I can still clearly remember just how great it felt to be able to cross my legs again with no assistance and showing this off at an OMS retreat!

With exercising it is possible to rewire the brain and relearn certain physical functions and movement thanks to the amazing neuroplasticity that exists in every brain at every age. It is possible to slow the loss of physical function and even recover some lost function regardless of age and where you are with the condition.

Look after the brain

Many with PMS will know what 'cog-fog' is. Forgetting words, losing track of what you're saying when you're speaking, not being able to concentrate or just not being able to think straight are all examples of this. And it's very normal to find this is worse when you're tired. The reason I had to stop working seven or so years after being diagnosed with PPMS was not because of physical problems (although they were there) but because I couldn't *think* well anymore—a bit of a bitter pill for someone with a PhD in quantum physics. Cognition issues can affect work relationships and also personal relationships—and more stressful conversations can be particularly difficult. Some may find that dealing with cognitive issues is actually more difficult than dealing with physical issues.

Loss of cognitive function and loss of grey matter in the brain are partly how the neurodegenerative component of MS presents itself. Exactly how these two are linked is still not clearly understood but it's both possible and important to protect and maintain your neurological reserve and your cognitive reserve. And as neurodegeneration is now acknowledged to be present in all forms of MS, this has led to the creation of the MS Brain Health initiative, chaired by Professor Gavin Giovannoni, looking at promoting the importance of brain health across all of the MS population.

How can cognitive reserve be protected and increased? As with other degenerative conditions, keeping the brain active is very important. Reading or learning something new like a new language or playing a musical instrument can help to protect against some of the cognitive symptoms of PMS. As with physical function, the brain has the capacity to improve cognitive functions through mental exercise obtained through intellectually stimulating activities. And there is now evidence that improving cognitive reserve may even slow loss of cognition over time.

Concentration issues are very common in people with PMS and this can be a hindrance to activities like reading. But, like many functions in the brain, we can actually teach ourselves to concentrate better, almost relearn how to concentrate. One of the benefits of a regular mindfulness practice is that it can improve concentration, yet another reason to meditate. Chapter 6 of this book by Associate Professor Craig Hassed, 'Meditation, mindfulness and the mind–body connection', provides more information on this.

Cognitive hobbies (like reading or painting or playing an instrument) can preserve and increase cognition and are linked to reduced cognitive impairment

In addition to protecting our cognition, there are things we can do that are neuroprotective and actually protect the brain itself. Exercise has been shown to protect the grey matter, and a healthy diet and not smoking can also play a part. Maintaining a healthy weight is also a factor, as is limiting the use of alcohol, and getting sufficient sleep.

Look after mental health

It is well established that there is a *causal* link between stress and exacerbation of MS symptoms, relapses and possibly even onset of the condition itself. Professor George Jelinek realised this over twenty years ago when he first developed the OMS approach, and recommended practising meditation as a means to help people with MS deal with stress more skilfully.

Depression and anxiety are very common in people with MS, even more so than in the general population and in people with other chronic conditions. The physiological response to anxiety and depression can cause the body to produce the same inflammatory reaction as the fight or flight response.

So it is important to look after mental health, just as much as it is to look after physical health. The 'journey' with PMS can be hard and mentally very difficult. Frequently dealing with 'new normal' and living with uncertainty needs courage, determination and mental strength.

The research into meditation, and particularly mindfulness, has exploded over the last few years, and both are discussed in Chapter 6. Mindfulness is now widely recommended for the general population as a treatment for anxiety and depression—and courses are even available in the United Kingdom through the National Health Service (NHS). Mindfulness is also being integrated into cognitive therapy and there is a 'third wave' of cognitive therapy called 'acceptance and commitment therapy' (ACT) designed specifically for people with long-term conditions.

So a regular meditation practice is strongly recommended for everyone with MS, and particularly for those with PMS. Just by meditating for short periods most days it is possible to learn how to switch on the 'relaxation response' and reduce levels of stress and anxiety. And many people with MS also find it helpful to consult a mental health specialist for additional support.

There are some additional benefits that can come from a deeper mindfulness practice that are particularly beneficial for people with PMS. Living with a condition where negative changes in function are common, and where this is less in our control, can be very challenging. The awareness of body, mind and self that comes from a deeper mindfulness meditation practice can make a tremendous difference. Mindfulness can help us become aware of our 'hard-wired' conditioned reactions, and once aware of these conditioned reactions, we can change them and literally rewire the brain to respond more skilfully to these changes and living with our 'new normal'. Pain is another common symptom of MS, and mindfulness has been shown to help with chronic pain.

Part of looking after mental health is how you relate to the condition. It's very normal for this to change quite dramatically, and understandably, over time. It's standard to be on a bit of an emotional rollercoaster ride following diagnosis—experiencing feelings of guilt, sadness, blame, anger and acceptance. The path is not linear and it is not necessarily sequential. And as your 'new normals' are likely to be ever changing, albeit slowly, this emotional journey may be one that you find yourself on many times as each new milestone is reached.

Look after mental health—it's as important as looking after physical health—so that you can live positively and well in the midst of changing physical and cognitive issues

Perhaps most importantly is that mindfulness can help to develop a much greater sense of kindness to oneself—and kindness really is at the core of mindfulness. It is the combined attitudes of kindness and gentleness, of courage and determination that provide the mental strength needed in living with a degenerative condition like PMS.

Live life
You are not alone
Living with a degenerative condition takes mental strength and resilience and having a 'community of support' to help on the journey is very important. For some the journey might be very difficult, but there is no need to undertake this journey alone. Having a good support network in place can make a huge difference and contribute strongly to resilience and mental strength. 'Community' is so important that it's perhaps worthy of being another key step within the OMS approach.

Family and friends typically form our closest support networks. But with a degenerative condition you may notice a change in some of these relationships. The implications of losing function may change the responsibilities within relationships, and this too is likely to have an impact. You may find some friendships and relationships get stronger and feel even more important, others less so.

Interacting and sharing experiences with other people with PMS, who really know what it is like to 'live a day in your shoes', can be reassuring and helpful. The OMS Circles are an excellent way to meet others with MS who have made or are making similar lifestyle choices and, probably more importantly, have made the choice to actively look after their own health and wellbeing.

Perhaps one of the good outcomes of the COVID-19 pandemic is the increased use of technology to communicate and an increase in interconnectedness across geography and demographics. So now it is possible to interact with like-minded people with MS from wherever you are in the world.

You don't need to do this on your own—get support from wherever you can. Living with a degenerative condition takes mental strength and resilience and having a community of support can be invaluable

Living with PMS will almost certainly involve working with MS professionals—including neurologists, MS nurses, neurological physiotherapists, continence specialists and a general practitioner. As this community is probably the 'gatekeeper' to new treatments and services, it is important to maintain these relationships. Chapter 11 of this book by Dr Heather King deals explicitly with choosing your medical team.

The different support networks can also help keep us aware of new and changing lifestyle interventions and options we have for *taking care of ourselves, and then help us act on our choices*. The OMS charity and other MS organisations regularly provide details of the latest research and evidence of treatments that may alter the trajectory of MS.

Identity and self

A diagnosis of PMS can have a profound impact on our identity and how we see ourselves. Just living with the uncertainty and unpredictability of the condition can be difficult and take time to adjust to. The different physical symptoms of PMS, such as walking difficulties, balance, fatigue, incontinence and pain, can hugely affect how we see ourselves. And these may lead to having to leave employment or stop doing hobbies and activities that are very important to the individual—my own worsening physical and mental functions resulted in me having to stop work and give up mountaineering, two activities that were incredibly important to me and, in my mind, largely defined who I was.

It can be a very helpful exercise to reflect on your *values* and what they are now—and these may or may not have changed very much since diagnosis. So what are values? There are lots of different ways these are defined, but they have been described as what you want to stand for in life, or the strengths and qualities that you want to develop or consider to be most important, or just what's most important to you. And values may be expressed in relation to various aspects of your life, such as family, personal relationships, hobbies, interests and work or livelihood.

PMS is likely to affect your identity, so use this as an opportunity to step back and reflect on who you are and what is important to you

After reflecting on values it can be useful to then think about what you do in your day-to-day life and try to align what you do with what's most important to you. It's unlikely that you'll be able to align everything you do with these values but if you manage to live at least some of life according to these values it can make a huge difference in terms of happiness and fulfillment.

Values may naturally change over time, so every year or so go back to your list of values and consider whether anything has changed. And if they have, then consider if you need or want to make any changes to your day-to-day life.

Take control and decide how to live life

Professor George Jelinek urges us in *Overcoming Multiple Sclerosis* to do whatever it takes to be well with MS, but what does this mean, particularly if you have the progressive form of the condition? Can we really affect the trajectory of the progressive form of MS?

In short, yes we can. Each of the lifestyle changes recommended in *Overcoming Multiple Sclerosis* can make a difference, while adopting them all compounds the effect, and some of the steps reinforce each other. Part of this is putting in place a mindset that we can 'take control' of our physical and mental health and that this will affect the PMS trajectory. So become your own health expert and keep abreast of new treatments and interventions.

This also includes taking control of your own mind and choosing how you want to respond to having this condition. This is perhaps one of the most important insights and realisations that I have taken from living with PMS for over thirteen years: that we can control how we respond to this condition and the changes it brings about. As Viktor Frankl famously said, 'Everything can be taken from a man or woman but one thing: the last of human freedoms—to choose one's attitude in any given set of circumstances, to choose one's own way.'

Understand what is important to you, do what you need to do and enjoy your unique life as it unfolds day by day

We can live rich and fulfilling lives with the progressive form of this condition. We may not know exactly how the condition will progress, as no individual knows how their life is going to unfold. But we can affect the trajectory of the condition. And what we can do is understand what is important to us, do what we need to do, and enjoy our unique life as it unfolds day by day.

Ground covered

Progressive MS (PMS) occurs in a smaller proportion of the MS population and typically results in the gradual loss of physical and cognitive function, although the rate of progression varies hugely between individuals, and in the majority, changes happen slowly over many years. Often PMS is presented as the 'most challenging' form of MS, partly because PMS is still poorly understood and there are very few treatments available.

There are lifestyle modifications that can protect the brain and neurological functions, and slow the rate of progression. The inherently 'plastic' nature of the brain and nervous system means that it is possible to restore and recover some lost function. So even with this seemingly inexorable form of the condition it is possible to take some control and affect the trajectory. PMS is different for everyone and recovery of function and improvements to progression will be different for us all.

Inevitably change will happen, and more so in some individuals than others. As with any degenerative condition, it is both the changes themselves and living with these 'new normals', and their impact on our lifestyles, employment and relationships, that make for challenges. Knowing that you can take some control of the trajectory of the condition and your own health can help build mental strength and resilience. Perhaps it can help you come to a better understanding of who you are and your own identity, so you can decide what to do to live life fully and in alignment with what's important for you.

My Story: Dave Jackman

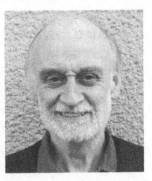

'You have primary progressive multiple sclerosis and I would expect someone in a similar position to need a walking stick in about three years and a wheelchair in another three.' Well, I did press my neurologist to be honest!

Nine years on, no walking stick or wheelchair in sight. I do like to remind him about the OMS Program during my annual reviews.

It was my wife Rae who, day one after diagnosis, discovered the work of Professor Swank, then on day three, found out about OMS. We really liked how the Program combined the longstanding evidence of Swank's work with more recent research-based findings around things like vitamin D and omega-3. More than anything it was evidence that we trusted and believed in. It gave us hope.

When we first had a look at the dietary changes, I know my wife had serious doubts as to whether I'd be able to change my lifestyle. I loved meat and dairy and was no fan of vegetables, but given the prognosis by my 'cheery' neurologist, I knew I had to try.

We started to follow the OMS lifestyle in November 2011. I kept a note of twelve symptoms I knew I had as a checklist.

For the next nine months, while following the OMS Program, many of my twelve symptoms deteriorated. However, after about a year I noticed that a few had stopped recurring, and while walking and balance were still (very) slowly deteriorating, the ten other symptoms improved and gradually disappeared.

In 2013 we attended the OMS Launde Abbey Retreat—the first one in the United Kingdom! Without being overdramatic, that week was life-changing.

Post retreat, I kept a log of the food I consumed and maintained my daily symptom checklist. I also visited a dietician to check out any intolerances I might have—dairy was a big one, plus celery and cats. Cats weren't a problem on a mainly vegan diet, though!

I normally walk 2–3 miles a day with our dog and I thought that was about my limit. Last year, Rae and I visited Padua in Italy and spent several days walking round this beautiful city. I was staggered to find that on day one I had walked 10 miles. Next day a mere 9. We reflected back to our first holiday plans after diagnosis when we thought a wheelchair would be needed to negotiate airports.

Rae and I enjoyed the Launde Abbey Retreat so much that we helped to organise a reunion the following year. And we've had more. Next year will be our seventh. We love meeting up with positive, like-minded people and return home feeling inspired, refreshed and with new ideas to try.

Notwithstanding MS, my health is better than ever. Rae and our family follow many aspects of the lifestyle and are heathier than they have ever been, too. Having an MS diagnosis really gave me a kickstart to adopting a much healthier lifestyle that I probably wouldn't have had the motivation to do otherwise. Now, where is that neurologist?

9

Families and prevention

Dr Sandra Neate and Dr Pia Jelinek

The lifestyle, the changes have benefited our relationship; it's definitely made us stronger because we both made the changes so we went through it together.

Natalie Harvey, South Africa, partner of person with MS and OMSer

Reading much of the medical information provided to people with MS or published in the scientific literature can be a depressing experience. MS is typically described as an illness causing progressive neurological decline and disability. It is rare to find any mention of what people with MS can do for themselves or any positive outcomes for them or their families. The future is often portrayed as bleak. As a result family members and others close to the person diagnosed with MS may experience worry, fear, anxiety and levels of stress that affect their own physical and mental health. Families face the question of what the diagnosis will mean not only for the person with MS, but the partner, the partnership and the family. Suffice to say, there is a lot that people can do to improve their own and their families' prospects for the future.

Partners
Partner experiences after a diagnosis of MS
Partners may experience feelings of loss and grief about the MS diagnosis and what it will mean for their lives. Difficult emotions

and frustrations can arise from day-to-day challenges. Uncertainty is an almost inevitable feature of living with MS as the course of the illness is often unpredictable. The more people feel uncertain about their futures, the more they experience the illness as interfering with their lives, setting up a vicious cycle. Having a sense of uncertainty interferes with planning simple things such as how to eat out or whether and where to travel, or may disrupt more major life decisions, such as planning families, careers and retirement.

Some couples develop a sense of urgency about decision-making, feeling they need to make important decisions while still fit and healthy. These include the decisions to have children, how many children to have, where to live and whether to change their working arrangements or retire. Others may feel so anxious or concerned about the future that they put off making decisions or they begin 'second guessing' their decisions, potentially making their feelings of uncertainty even worse.

However, there is a new paradigm emerging around more positive experiences, based on people with MS committing to lifestyle changes that offer real potential for better health and more stable long-term outcomes. Improved outcomes may provide a new sense of hope for the future and replace feelings of fear and uncertainty. Finding hope for a positive future early after diagnosis can literally change the outlook for people with MS and their partners, whose decisions may well be more balanced.

Hope is a powerful antidote to uncertainty, both for people with MS and their partners

Are there any benefits to living with MS?

Now for the good news. Couples living with MS almost universally experience what is termed adversarial growth—that is, they experience personal growth through facing the challenges that the illness presents. Interestingly, the growth for each member of the couple does not relate to the seriousness of the challenges they face. Rather, what affects whether the partner experiences growth is whether the person with MS has a growth experience and vice versa, an

For many partners, MS provides opportunities; paradoxically it may offer some new choices

interesting interdependence between the partner and the person with MS. Making choices and dealing with challenges together obviously play a major role in how the couple grows.

Many partners also recount that MS provides an opportunity for them to re-evaluate their lives and to re-prioritise what is important to them, individually and as a couple. This is a common theme following any life-changing event. Many partners and couples report gratitude for the chance that dealing with MS provides to take stock of their busy lives and re-examine their careers, friendships, lifestyle choices, even where they live. The sense of urgency to make decisions based on uncertainty is replaced by an urge to take steps to make positive change and to reframe attitudes to see change as a challenge that will strengthen them individually and as a couple.

Can changing lifestyle benefit the relationship?

And there is more good news. Extensive research has found that the modification of lifestyle-related risk factors for MS, such as diet, exercise, supplementation with vitamin D and omega-3 oils and stress-reduction techniques, as described in this book, has been associated with significantly improved outcomes for people with MS. Improved outcomes include decreased fatigue, decreased relapse rate and risk of depression and decreased risk of worsening disability. Most importantly, quality of life—that is, one's day-to-day experience of life—is significantly better. This improvement applies both to the health of the body and the mind—in other words, to physical and mental health. And, after all, what is more important than one's experience of life?

And of great interest to partners is another level of interconnectedness between the members of the couple. The partner's quality of life directly relates to the health of the person with MS and how that person feels about their health. And very importantly, the partner's quality of life is more dependent on the *mental health* of the person with MS than on their physical health. So if the person with MS feels better about themselves and experiences less depression, their partner will also experience a better quality of life. Not surprising, really! If the physical and mental health improves for the person with MS, so will that of their partner.

The wellbeing of a person with MS is dependent on the wellbeing of their partner and vice versa

So it makes sense that the adoption of healthy lifestyle behaviours by people with MS can improve the health of their partners. It becomes increasingly clear that the health and quality of life of the individuals within the relationship are highly dependent on each other and health may prosper for each if improved outcomes are experienced.

How can a partner support lifestyle modification?

A partner can provide support in many ways. Each partner will make their own decisions and decide what feels right for them. Support may take a very practical form, such as shopping for and preparing meals, providing time and space for meditation or supporting and encouraging the person's exercise-related activities. Some partners decide to 'keep the home fires burning' and provide a supportive environment for the person with MS to undertake change, lessening the sense for the person with MS that they are dealing with this alone.

Others might undertake quite extensive research and read widely to understand the OMS Program and other research regarding MS, providing a kind of translation role for the person with MS, who may be busy dealing with more practical issues. This 'buying in' is in distinct contrast to denial, where both partners bury their heads in the sand, leading to worse outcomes for health and the relationship.

Others may choose to undertake changes themselves. Once again, this may provide a practical benefit. Preparing and sharing the same meals may make mealtime simpler than if the family is eating different meals, but either can work. Exercising and meditating together adds a further dimension to these activities and many partners report the great benefits of enjoyment of undertaking new activities together.

The motivation for and degree of change undertaken by the partner may evolve over time as partners consider and evaluate their own needs and health imperatives and make personal choices regarding their degree of engagement with lifestyle modification.

Partners and family can enjoy unexpected benefits to their own health through adopting the lifestyle changes that the person with MS makes

The dynamics of each relationship vary and the individual partner has their life as a couple and as an individual to deal with. Everyone must find what is right for them.

For a partner who undertakes lifestyle modification themselves, together with the person with MS, the advantages can be quite significant. As already mentioned, the partner's quality of life may be improved simply due to the mental and physical health benefits to the person with MS. But many partners who have adopted change report much more than this, and they notice significant improvements to their own health and the health of their families, through dietary modification, increased physical activity and stress-reduction techniques. And not to forget that partners and children are not immune from health problems of their own and need to look after themselves!

Advantages of adoption of lifestyle modification as a couple

Apart from the health benefits, partners may experience a wealth of less tangible or obvious benefits. The adoption of lifestyle modification may give the couple a sense of control of their health. Self-management—that is, taking responsibility for one's own choices and undertaking behaviours that will enhance health and wellbeing—is a concept of increasing interest and importance in the strategies for management of chronic illness across the board in medicine. It emphasises the individual's responsibility for managing their own health, and also incorporates the positive contribution of family, community and the medical profession. It is a change from the model where doctors provide advice and patients receive the information in a passive manner. Self-management aims to encourage and inspire individuals to actively identify challenges and solve problems associated with the illness for themselves.

The knowledge and evidence-based information provided through the OMS Program allows couples to undertake self-management, to make informed, rational choices regarding treatments and how they will live their lives. After taking on lifestyle modification, some partners have described enjoying feeling that 'MS doesn't control us anymore. We control the MS'. They develop a sense of teamwork, enjoy the joint decision-making and experience feelings of empowerment.

Lifestyle modification may lead to a sense of mastery and hope, and optimism may follow

This sense of control and empowerment that comes with undertaking proactive changes is often described as developing a sense of mastery. Having mastery diminishes the feeling of uncertainty that can plague the couple. For those who actually experience improvements in physical and mental health and develop mastery, hope along with optimism and confidence are likely to arise. Hope and optimism about the future are often the first casualties of a serious life-altering diagnosis.

New and other partnerships

Much of the previous information relates to established intimate partnerships. But what about those people with MS venturing into and establishing new relationships? People with MS may experience feelings of low self-worth and worry when diagnosed that they may be a burden to those in a future relationship. Given many of the findings around improved outcomes for those undertaking lifestyle modification, people embarking on new relationships could view them as an opportunity to make choices that support their health and wellbeing. People with MS and their partners can have confidence that there is potential for strong, enduring relationships where couples embrace self-management techniques. There is also the potential within relationships for the exploration of things that would never have otherwise been experienced.

Naturally there are many varieties of important relationships that can exist other than intimate relationships. People with MS can be supported by other family members, friends or mentors. Such relationships can be of great importance and can provide practical and emotional support and inspiration to the person with MS. As with intimate partnerships these relationships can also be strengthened and benefit from the shared experience of MS.

Children

When faced with a diagnosis of MS, many people's thoughts turn immediately to their children. How will I tell them? How will they react? Will I be a burden to my children? Will they develop MS?

Telling children about MS

Naturally this is a personal decision for all couples. When the time feels right, discussing the issue in an age-appropriate and honest way is vital. The idea of protecting children by not telling them about the diagnosis, or 'sugar coating' it, frequently leads to children expressing resentments later in life. Children may feel let down that they weren't trusted with being able to cope, or worse, that they couldn't help because they didn't know the situation. There is clearly a cost to secrecy. Initially, of course, it may be wise to allow a little time to plan how and what to tell the children, and to let the difficult emotions around diagnosis settle a little.

Children have a good radar for not being told the truth and generally appreciate honesty

Interestingly, again, the mental health outcomes of children of people with MS depend mainly on the mental health of their parents and the adjustment and functioning of the family. Across the board, independent of disease duration or disability, children of people with MS have similar educational outcomes, development and ability to establish and maintain relationships as other children. The most important thing for children to flourish is open and clear communication. The recipe for success is that children need to be well informed and to maintain a balance between care and concern for the parent and realising their own goals.

Should children undertake lifestyle modification?

Once again, every family is different and the needs of family members and children should be considered. Some children's needs may even exceed that of the person with MS. As we have said, self-management is an important strategy for illness prevention. This can be extrapolated to management of the health of children from an early age. By establishing a pattern for taking responsibility for one's own health early in life and providing strategies for mitigating illness and managing it in later life, children's health is likely to be positively affected by lifestyle changes and the 'dinner table' conversations that surround these changes.

Parents may feel guilty that their children are missing out or being burdened in some way but providing them with the knowledge and tools to understand their own risks and make their own choices is by no means a burden. As with partners, all children must eventually find their own way, and of course, later in life will make their own choices. Every person has their own health imperatives, and while those of the children may not be as pressing as those of their parent, they may choose many differing ways of managing their own lives, and should be encouraged to do so. Children who undertake lifestyle modification may also substantially reduce their risk of developing MS, to which we know they are particularly susceptible.

Preventing MS in family members

A diagnosis of MS for a family member may be a very difficult experience, in similar but also different ways from that of a partner. Having a parent, child, sibling, member of the extended family or even an in-law diagnosed with MS can be a life-changing event for the entire family.

Having a family member with MS increases a person's risk of getting MS themselves. This risk depends on how closely related the two individuals are. Knowing that they have a higher chance of receiving the same diagnosis and following the same path as their family member can be confronting. The good news is that the risk to family members may be substantially reduced through a number of targeted lifestyle changes.

Family members' risk of developing MS

Children, siblings and even parents of people with MS are at a greater risk of developing MS. All relatives have a higher risk of MS, but some are at greater risk than others. The general population has around a 1 in 300 to 1 in 1000 chance of developing MS, depending on where you live. The risk for an immediate (first-degree) family member, again varying considerably with location, is about one in ten. This risk increases with the number of relatives with MS that a person has. Another way of thinking about this is that MS is said to be up to 20–40 times more likely if one has a brother, sister, child or parent with the disease, depending on that person's other environmental circumstances. That's a big increase in risk, and a very good reason to consider the ways in which we can reduce these numbers.

Close relatives of people with MS are at an increased risk of developing MS themselves

When thinking about risk, it is often helpful to think about identical twins. In this context, if an identical twin has MS the other twin has about a one in four chance of developing the disease. Of course, there are other environmental factors that increase the risk too, such as smoking, which doubles the risk of MS, or low vitamin D levels, and these are clearly more important than the genetic risk as they account for the other three-quarters of the risk. These are the factors that can be changed, and thus the factors that we want to focus our attention on.

Can a family member alter their risk?

Recognising this increased risk in family members presents a golden opportunity to make changes to ensure that the risk is minimised. The good

Family members can benefit generally from healthy lifestyle changes, but these changes can also reduce their chances of getting MS

news is that there are a number of simple lifestyle changes a family member of someone with MS can make to reduce their chance of getting MS, even when their baseline risk is higher than most.

Quit smoking

Avoiding both smoking and other people's cigarette smoke is crucial for close relatives of people with MS. A person who smokes is roughly one and a half to two times more likely to develop MS than a non-smoker. Children are also more likely to develop MS if their parents smoke. The longer the child is exposed to the cigarette smoke, the more likely MS is to develop. Children are also more likely to adopt behaviours modelled by their parents. If a child does take up smoking, they are then at an even higher risk.

Smoking has a detrimental effect for people with MS, both in terms of disability and quality of life. If a person is more disabled and has a worse quality of life, one can imagine the effect this might have on the people around them. Quitting smoking is one of the most important and effective steps in reducing the risk of MS in close relatives. If anyone in the family quits, the benefits are far-reaching, beyond just those they will personally experience.

Get adequate sun exposure regularly

The risk of MS is considerably reduced for those family members who receive adequate sun exposure. There are benefits of sun exposure beyond reducing MS risk, as one might imagine. Getting outdoors is generally good for the body, mind and soul. Doing this with minimal clothing on in order to maximise sun exposure and vitamin D synthesis is even better. For details regarding safe, adequate sun exposure, see Chapter 4 by Dr Conor Kerley. The recommended amount of sun exposure for people with MS and their families is the same: that is, 10–15 minutes of as close to all-over sun exposure as possible on a day where the UV index is 7 3–5 times a week.

Supplement with vitamin D

Taking a vitamin D supplement at an adequate dose has been shown to be associated with reduced risk of MS developing in relatives of people with MS. Immediate family members should take 5000 IU of vitamin D3 daily in winter and on days when sun exposure in summer is limited. This dose should be appropriately reduced for children, so a child of say eight years of age who weighs 25 kilograms should take 2500 IU a day. At this sort of dosage, blood-level monitoring of vitamin D is not required, although it might be prudent to have it checked every few years.

Vitamin D supplementation should be routine in pregnancy, just as folic acid is, and reduces the risk of MS for the newborn. All at-risk children—that is, those who are in a family in which someone has MS—should take vitamin D supplements. Taking vitamin D is a practical and cost-effective way of protecting families, and, on a broader scale, reducing the incidence of MS in the world. The dose that we recommend for family members is somewhat lower than the dose we recommend for people with MS as the minimum blood level required for prevention is not as high as for those with the illness and this avoids the need for regular blood testing. For relatives, we recommend aiming for a blood level of above 100 nmol/L; however, levels anywhere up to 225 nmol/L (90 mcg/mL in the United States) are quite safe and within the normal range. The benefits go well beyond reducing the risk of developing MS; vitamin D can improve mood, quality of life, immune function and bone health, and reduce risk of other chronic Western diseases such as heart disease.

Eat a healthy diet low in saturated fat

The evidence is not quite so clear-cut whether family members choosing to eat the same diet as the person with MS will reduce their risk. This is where it is useful to think about risk versus benefits. What are the risks of going on such a diet? Are there any side effects? Many people ask about vitamin and mineral deficiencies from eating a diet that is plant-based. They are in fact exceedingly rare. The OMS diet is a plentiful source of the important vitamins and minerals.

On the other hand, what are the potential benefits of family members going on the OMS diet? Professor Roy Swank writes in *The Multiple Sclerosis Diet Book* (2nd edition, 1987) about how he placed all the family members of 3,500 people with MS on the same diet. He tracked them over decades, and found that not one of their relatives on the diet developed the disease.

It is also known that following a generally healthy diet with more fruit, vegetables and wholefoods and fewer animal products, processed foods and saturated fat is important in preventing many other chronic health conditions such as heart disease and type 2 diabetes. Another great benefit of having families eat the same healthy diet is that their chances of developing these conditions also decreases.

Supplement with flaxseed oil

Consuming flaxseed oil regularly is associated with a lower risk of developing MS. In fact, regularly taking flaxseed oil (the most potent plant-based omega-3 fatty acid) as part of our diet could reduce the risk of MS by up to 40 per cent! Practically, taking fresh flaxseed oil is the best way to ingest omega-3 fatty acids. Fish oil is not as good and has not actually been shown to provide any benefit at all. Flaxseed oil is another one of those recommendations that has lots of other great side effects; in this case it lowers cholesterol, prevents heart disease and helps to prevent inflammatory illnesses. The recommendation is to take 20–40 millilitres per day as food—that is, poured over meals just before eating them. After a while, one realises that there is no need to measure; a liberal splash over food is perfect!

Keep stress levels down with meditation and mindfulness
Mindfulness-based stress reduction or meditation is a key step in the prevention of MS. It is about sitting with oneself on a regular basis for a defined period of time and allowing what's there to be there and simply observing it, without judgement.

You may be surprised to discover the myriad benefits that mindfulness provides, as outlined in Chapter 6. Mindfulness meditation is an approved first-line treatment for depression in the United Kingdom and we know it improves overall quality of life. It is one of only two interventions that exists that actually grows new brain cells in the areas of the brain that are important to higher executive function and shrinks the parts of the brain that are unhelpful (the other intervention is exercise, which will be looked at next). Mindfulness-based stress reduction reduces pain, increases compassion and resilience, and reduces reactivity to difficult situations. This is just the tip of the iceberg of the benefits of mindfulness, which are discussed more in depth in Chapter 6. So, there are literally no downsides to searching for a guided meditation on the OMS website and giving it a go.

To reduce the risk of developing MS, family members should quit smoking, get adequate sun exposure, supplement with vitamin D and flaxseed oil, practise mindfulness and exercise

Exercise regularly
The vast benefits of exercise are well known. In general, people are healthier and happier when they exercise regularly. Everyone, everywhere should exercise in whatever way they can. Any exercise is better than none. It is as simple as that.

Regular exercise is likely to help protect relatives who do not show signs of MS. And the best thing about exercise is that there are no negative side effects! It is very probable that not only will the risk of MS go down, but we may become generally healthier and happier people.

How can my family make these changes?

Simply placing all family members on the same diet may not be as easy as it sounds. Instead, it may be easiest to start with the more simple and pleasurable interventions for the less-motivated family members, such as increasing sun exposure. Just getting families outdoors in the sunshine can have a hugely valuable effect on quality of life and play a vital role in preventing MS. Similarly, taking a vitamin D supplement is quick, easy, cheap and effective, and may be easier to accept in the initial stages than a major change in diet or activity. There are even tasty, chewable vitamin D supplements available for little ones!

It doesn't really matter where you start, but vitamin D supplementation is a simple and easy addition to most people's lives and a good place to begin changing the family routine

Quitting smoking is undoubtedly difficult. For many people it is a habit that has formed over many years, so deeply ingrained that they may struggle to imagine life without it. Remember that the majority of smokers quit without the need for medication or any other help. Around 75 per cent of people simply quit, cold turkey; it is by far the most successful way to quit. It is also important to remember that many people try and fail. This is normal. The old adage 'if at first you don't succeed, try, try again' is particularly pertinent here.

Other benefits for family members from adopting lifestyle modifications

As with partners adopting change, if all family members, especially those living together, take on the lifestyle modifications, the advantages can be more than just health-related. It is much more convenient to make one dinner for the entire family. Getting outdoors and doing exercise together as a family can be an enjoyable bonding experience.

Some family members may find it difficult to accept and implement some or all of these adjustments to their life. If very young, it might be difficult to understand why these changes are occurring and why they are necessary. Barriers to change are common and often require some time to address. Time may also be required to adapt practically to the new routine—for instance, changing the common habit of eating meals based on meat. It will be easier to adjust to the new normal of creating plant-based meals that the whole family can enjoy if everyone is on the same page with a common goal in mind.

Adopting lifestyle modifications as a family can be convenient and provide an opportunity for family bonding

Having the entire family take on the same changes can also be helpful for the affected family member. Tackling the challenges together often brings families closer and creates a more supportive environment. Large family gatherings may start to look a little different. Support from the extended family can be important and beneficial for everybody.

While some family members may welcome education and encouragement to adopt these lifestyle interventions, certain family members may not wish to be involved in some or all of the lifestyle modifications; they might not be ready to talk openly, nor accept changes in their own life. They also require support. Every individual needs to find their own way.

Community

After a person is diagnosed with MS, partners and families may also experience less social interaction. Social support is one of the few things known to directly positively influence the health of partners. So it's important for partners of people with MS to maintain a strong social network. Social connection through friends, family, groups, health practitioners and online communities like the OMS Forum (see the OMS website, overcomingms.org) may provide significant benefit. Other family members should be encouraged to maintain existing social circles as a valuable form of emotional support and use available communities and groups and other external sources, outside the family unit.

Ground covered

The effects of a diagnosis of MS on the lives of partners, family and friends are not to be underestimated. In the past there has been a lot of focus on the negative effects, with deterioration of relationships often occurring in parallel with personal health deterioration for the person with the illness. But it doesn't have to be this way. If the person with MS takes some control, gets a sense of hope, purpose and confidence back, through developing a plan to change lifestyle for the better, then the effects on those around them can be profound. More importantly, a shared sense of control through partner support, particularly through the partner personally adopting some or all of the changes, can strengthen relationships and make for a stable, confident future for all involved.

As MS is a disease that runs in families, people with MS are often concerned about the future of their close relatives. Fortunately, there are many lifestyle changes that relatives can make that have been shown to be associated with decreased risk. The changes made by other family members may reduce risk, improve health and demonstrate support to the person with MS and the whole family unit.

My Story:
Leah Tsirigotis

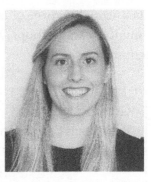

I remember being aware of MS from a young age. I'd grown up knowing two family friends who had MS, and recall asking my mum when I was quite young why one of them always had his 'shepherd's crook' with him. Eventually he swapped the crook for more frequent use of his wheelchair before I inevitably stopped seeing him as his declining mobility made it difficult for him to leave the house.

This flashback came immediately flooding back to me when my husband Alex called me late on a Thursday night in June 2013 (while I was five months pregnant), letting me know the verdict from his follow-up MRI scan appointment. His neurologist had diagnosed him with MS.

It was a huge shock for both of us. I'd known he had issues with blurred vision, balance and at times brain fog but I'd thought it more akin to him having a visual migraine . . . not MS. The outlook presented to us by the neurologist on follow up seemed grim: three years until significant mobility issues and an initial suspicion of primary progressive multiple sclerosis (PPMS).

Determined to avoid a quick decline, we spent a lot of time researching. Within three days we had looked through several programs of living with MS and settled on the OMS Program as a first step. We ordered two books by Prof Jelinek (*Overcoming Multiple Sclerosis: The evidence-based 7 step recovery program* [2nd edn, 2016] and *Recovering From Multiple Sclerosis: Real life stories of hope and inspiration* [2013]) and before they'd even arrived Alex had started making the dietary changes and incorporating meditation into his daily routine. About a month later we had all his trousers and shorts adjusted to accommodate the weight loss!

Knowing that there was an elevated risk to close family members (siblings, children, and so on) of someone with MS, as discussed in *Overcoming Multiple Sclerosis*, I'm grateful we received Alex's diagnosis and found the OMS Program prior to having our first child. The research that we read about preventing family members from getting MS made adoption of the OMS Program (diet, vitamin D, exercise and meditation) for the whole family, from birth, a natural step for us.

Several years on, there has thankfully been little progression in Alex's condition. There are times when he has an episode of vision loss, mainly when running (which, fortunately, he is able to do a lot of) and on occasion experiences stress-induced brain fog (who doesn't?). His suspected diagnosis of PPMS was revised by his neurologist a few months after diagnosis to relapsing remitting MS, and after seven years on the OMS Program I'm pleased to say he is free of mobility problems. He has discovered a love of ultra-running and the kids and I have developed a love of supporting him in his endeavours and at times even joining in with them.

For us the OMS Program shone a light of hope when we truly believed there would be none and opened a door to a community of people going through different stages of their individual journeys with MS. It gave us both confidence that we could do more than wait for progression to happen and allowed us (over time) to be less afraid of the future. Now, as a family of four, we are proud members of a large running and natural-living community, and are excited for the future.

I could not be more grateful to the amazing start we had with the OMS Program on our recovery journey.

Part 3

Keeping on track

10

I've just been diagnosed with MS

Dr Sam Gartland

On reflection, my diagnosis of MS has allowed me to strengthen my resolve in all aspects of my health, thoughts and actions.

Andrea Jelleff, Melbourne, Australia, OMSer

'It's bad news, you've got MS.' I shook my head, not wanting to hear the news. I'd been sure for some time that this was the case, but I'd been trying to ignore it. It had begun with incredible fatigue. I'd been low on energy and struggling to make it into work for some time. I remember arriving at work and finding it remarkable how fresh and light my colleagues looked. I'd literally have to summon all my will to get out of bed and make it into work. Then I developed the numbness in my legs and the tell-tale Lhermitte's sign (the electric shock–type sensation that passes down the back of your neck and into your spine) and I knew what the issue was. However, I had important professional exams coming up and getting ill, now, really didn't fit in with my plans. But I'd become very sick and when it was obvious that I couldn't walk from the car park to the intensive care unit I was working in, a colleague examined me and arranged an urgent MRI scan.

I was given the news by a kind but direct surgeon I knew. While I was initially distressed, his initial comment was, 'Well at least it's not a brain tumour.' I remember thinking: *Yes, that's a fair comment.*

The following day I went to see the neurologist, and my wife came along to support me. He mentioned that 'some people find dietary changes help' but that the evidence wasn't strong. I didn't register this at the time but my wife picked up on it and has since reminded me.

Given that I had only had one episode and some 'non-specific' lesions on the brain scan, it was agreed that we wouldn't call this MS but rather a clinically isolated syndrome (CIS) and I would remain under review.

I had some time off to recuperate and my mind was mixed up—as was my course of action. My initial response had been to go to the pub to numb the shock with alcohol. Other responses were more helpful. I felt drawn to nature as it felt healing. I've since learned that this is a common reaction for many when illness occurs. I went for walks in the countryside, made an effort to get some sun and took the opportunity to exercise more. As a student I had exercised and meditated regularly. This had slipped when I began work as a junior doctor. Part of me remained in denial.

A colleague had told me about Professor Jelinek's book *Taking Control of Multiple Sclerosis*, and I found the information compelling, but my diagnosis was still 'uncertain'. I hadn't felt that I needed to radically change my life yet. I remember thinking, just one more relapse, like an optic neuritis, and I will make the changes required.

I went back to my usual pattern of life and during my first night back on call I had a relapse. It came on quickly and suddenly. I was on my own anaesthetising at night when my eyesight went. I now knew there was no doubt. This time I came away with my mind in a mess. For all the reasoned science in the *Taking Control of Multiple Sclerosis* book, my mind fell back to what I'd seen of MS. I had seen young people, especially men, deteriorate rapidly. Surely if simply changing your diet could halt this illness, the neurologists would have been recommending this to all their patients? Diet and lifestyle interventions in MS had never been mentioned in my training.

It was around this time that the head of my specialist training scheme contacted me by text saying that he would countersign the forms so that I could retire from work due to ill health. I was 32. The next few months are a bit of a blur now. It was turning into winter in the north of England and the days were cold and short. I sat at home with my mind racing with thoughts of sadness, anger and frustration. I remember a visit from my MS nurse to show me how to use the injectable medicine Copaxone. This and steroid tablets were all the treatment that I was offered. I remember looking at the small vials and thinking that this was a completely inadequate response to the challenge I was facing. I asked whether, in her experience, she thought my career in medicine was over—she said yes.

While sitting at home ruminating on my situation I fell into behaviours that distracted me from my predicament but did not always serve me well. At times these were unproductive and caused distress to those I cared about. There is a reason that pubs, bottle shops, bookmakers and the like are so common in Western societies. We seek escape from our suffering and if we haven't developed good coping strategies it is easy to compound our problems.

I had been in regular contact with friends and family during this time. I had mentioned Professor Jelinek's book and the potential to take control of this disease. I am fortunate that my parents discussed this with me and made sure I booked into the next retreat as a matter of urgency.

In January 2009 I flew out to Melbourne with my wife and attended the retreat at the Gawler Foundation. I remember seeing George and immediately noticed how well and vibrant he looked. I now *believed* that you could be well following the diagnosis of MS. That week was probably the most important week of my life (as I know it has been for many others). I found the meditation and sessions on emotional healing particularly helpful. It allowed me to let go of the emotions and distress that I was holding on to and be able to move to a mental space in which my energies would now be focused on doing whatever it took to be well.

On returning to the United Kingdom I applied for a new job that would allow me the time that I needed for self-care. I had previously qualified as a general practitioner (primary care physician) and I managed to get a job for two days a week with a long break in the day to allow me to rest. I'm disappointed to say that getting this job wasn't straightforward. I had at least two instances of job offers being withdrawn when my MS diagnosis came to light. There were and are legal protections in place, but I didn't have the desire to fight any more battles.

I used the time outside of work to grow and develop. I meditated regularly, sought the help of a clinical psychologist and began a yoga practice. Over the course of the next twelve months I got back to full-time work. I knew I wanted to live closer to nature and be in a better climate with more sun and I was fortunate to be able to move to Australia. During this time I enjoyed the incredible support of my wife, Lisette, our families and close friends. I remain forever grateful for and mindful of the support I was given at such a difficult time.

Responding to the diagnosis of MS

I recount the details of my own story here as the themes it covers will be familiar to all of us affected by this disease. Receiving a diagnosis of MS is a shocking and frightening experience. Most will recognise the feelings of grief, fear, anger, denial and maybe even relief that accompanies this news. There is often a reluctance to initially confirm the diagnosis, both on the part of the people with MS but often also their (well-meaning) doctors. This can be a collusion in denial and may prevent us from taking the action that is required.

After a diagnosis of MS our doctors often collude with us in our denial

But our reactions and the decisions that we make in response to this news end up determining the course of the disease and the long-term consequences that it has for us and those we care about. It is critical therefore to express emotions, accept the difficulties that this diagnosis presents and respond constructively. It is not a smooth path and there are difficulties along the way. We find ourselves moving to a new life and leaving our pre-MS life behind. We need to embrace this, as the path we were previously on made us sick in the first place. The steps of the OMS Program represent the path back to good health. Doing this with the support of friends and family makes the process much easier.

Our planned destination is good health

Contrary to what many people with MS are told, MS is not an enigma. We have very good knowledge of the causes of MS and what affects the course of the disease. It is similar to the other Western chronic medical conditions, in that it is mainly due to lifestyle factors. We are fortunate that now there is a clear roadmap of what is required to stabilise and even reverse this condition.

In the first few months after diagnosis there is a lot of information to take in and some of the information and advice available can be confusing and contradictory. Unfortunately, many people with MS are still not given that most basic and essential bit of information: MS is a disease largely due to lifestyle factors and the course of MS is nearly entirely due to these.

The *Journal of Neurology* made clear in a January 2018 editorial that 'encouraging a healthy lifestyle (healthy eating, a normal weight, routine physical activity and avoiding smoking) should be a fundamental message we give to all newly diagnosed patients with MS'.

This statement appeared nearly twenty years after the basis of the OMS Program was established. Since then, the supporting evidence for the Program has become stronger and people with MS can be confident that the OMS Program offers a reliable and detailed approach to guide our journey back to health. None of the steps are removed from general public health guidelines and all are straightforward to follow. It just requires a commitment to ourselves to become informed, put ourselves first and make the changes necessary for us to return to good health.

I'm now embarrassed to write that I hadn't appreciated the importance of diet and lifestyle when I was diagnosed—though this is a common oversight of many doctors and reflects our lack of training in nutrition. It is not uncommon for medical professionals to be slow to communicate basic health information to the public. The dangers of smoking were recognised as early as the late 1800s. It wasn't until 1964 (and more than 7000 scientific papers confirming the link) that the US Surgeon General warned the public of the dangers of smoking. Even then the American Medical Association wouldn't endorse the message (having just received $10 million from the tobacco companies). When it comes to our health and the advice we receive from our doctors there are many influences at play.

'To solve a problem you need to remove the cause, not the symptom.'—Liezi

What is health? The World Health Organization definition of health is 'a state of complete physical, mental and social well-being and not merely the absence of disease or infirmity'.

Therefore, we can see that we aren't simply aiming to 'treat MS'. We can use this opportunity to re-evaluate all aspects of our lives and restore balance to give us the best opportunity of living long lives, free of the common burdens of Western disease.

Roadmap for the first few months

In the box on the following page I outline in dot-point format the steps that I believe form the basis of setting out on the road to recovery after a diagnosis of MS. Of course, everyone will be different in the exact details of whatever approach they adopt. I bring to this my training in medicine and years of managing a variety of medical conditions in general practice. But more importantly, I bring my own experience of the diagnosis of MS and my own recovery. The outline I provide is a useful one to follow. Why? Because the science, my medical training and experience, and my personal experience of MS show that it works!

- Work through the adjustment reaction of being diagnosed with MS; express the grief and move on to take up the challenge of MS.
- Take time out to allow yourself to recuperate and begin the process of change and recovery; connect with your authentic self.
- Set the intention that you are going to stabilise this condition; commit to doing whatever it takes and to enjoy doing this.
- Educate yourself about the causes of MS and what exacerbates the condition; read the *Overcoming Multiple Sclerosis* book, attend an OMS workshop or education seminar and engage with the OMS Forum.
- Inform friends and family of your new lifestyle and why you are implementing it.
- Start your journey through the OMS Program.
- If you smoke, stop!
- Consider disease-modifying therapies (medications) if necessary.
- Ensure your vitamin D level is in the right range.
- Join a meditation group; learn about plant-based wholefood cooking, try new foods.
- Join some different exercise classes.
- Monitor your progress, consider writing a journal, commit to resolving 'disease'.
- Stay connected; maintain contact with friends and family; commit time to be with people you care about; build and cultivate your support networks.

Reviewing our beliefs and behaviours

As we have seen it is essential to work through the emotions following the diagnosis of MS and move forward to constructively engage with the challenge. We can release these feelings in many ways: through writing, such as keeping a journal, through music or

*An important
initial step is to get
rid of unhelpful
thought patterns
and behaviours
that are likely
to impede our
progress towards
recovery*

speaking with friends and loved ones, seeing a therapist and joining support groups. It is crucial to allow these emotions to be released. It allows us to move on to making the changes needed to recover from MS. This process of releasing emotions is also likely to have a beneficial impact on the disease process. The simple process of writing about a difficult life experience has been shown to reduce disease activity by 30 per cent in rheumatoid arthritis (like MS it is an autoimmune inflammatory disorder).

Many people with MS will find it helpful to engage the services of a psychologist or counsellor for therapies like cognitive behaviour therapy (CBT). CBT specifically addresses patterns of thinking and behaviour. By reviewing our thoughts and beliefs it is possible to change our attitudes and behaviours. We are then able to move forward to a new life relatively free of the patterns that have led to this illness. These are replaced by new beliefs, choices and actions that begin the process of stabilisation and recovery. We know that people with MS who do this have significantly better quality of life and outcomes. Speak with your treating healthcare providers about this. They will know of the good practitioners in your area and ways to access them.

For more information on mental health support see Chapter 12 on mental health by Dr Keryn Taylor, and Chapter 13 on resilience by Dr Rachael Hunter and also Chapter 6 on meditation and mindfulness by Associate Professor Craig Hassed.

Empowerment (self-efficacy or mastery)

This is a process and outcome whereby people can gain control over their own health. People with MS who take an active role in their care generally have improved outcomes and overall better quality of life. For this to occur three things are required:

1. autonomy—our actions need to be of our choosing and based on our thoughts and beliefs
2. competence—we need to feel capable of performing the actions required to achieve the outcome we are aiming for
3. relatedness—we need to care about others and to feel cared for by others.

So, we can see that if we understand that MS and its progression are largely due to lifestyle and environmental factors, then, if we wish to be well, we know that we need to assert our *autonomy*, take control and choose to optimise those factors known to be risk factors for the progression of MS, and develop the competence needed and the relationships required to support these changes.

Known risk factors for the development of MS that are thought to be involved in its progression as well are described in detail in other chapters and include a Western diet high in saturated fats and low in omega-3 fats, consumption of cow's milk, low vitamin D levels in the blood and low sun exposure, smoking, stress and our reactions to it, including depression, and viral infections (e.g. Epstein Barr virus, human herpes virus). Importantly, we have control over all of these apart from our exposure to viral infections.

To become *competent* to make these changes we need to develop and grow. This may include harnessing the resources from the OMS Program. It can also mean seeking inspiration and help from many other sources, and in that process learning from other positive stories of recovery. Developing new skills like meditation and mindfulness, taking part in new sports and activities, discovering new things to cook and eat, making new friends and social connections: these are all highly desirable actions that in turn can increase our relatedness. It becomes a virtuous cycle.

The importance of *relatedness* and social support cannot be overstated. Feeling loved and cared for at a challenging time is of great help. When you have friends and family supporting you it makes life much easier. They can support us in our food and lifestyle choices. They can help with practical matters such as attending healthcare appointments and dealing with administrative tasks.

As well as the practical benefits of maintaining a good social network, it has also been shown to improve physical and mental health, help maintain brain health, reduce inflammation, speed up recovery from major illness and prolong lifespan.

In the early days following the diagnosis there is a lot to take in. It is known that even under optimal circumstances much information from appointments with doctors isn't correctly recalled. A support person is likely to improve recall of what has been discussed and agreed at the appointment.

Take time to read about proposed treatments. Reliable resources include the OMS website, MS Australia and the MS Trust. It is appropriate to read up on your proposed treatment and agree on a plan with your treating team. Don't feel rushed into treatment decisions and have the confidence to raise questions. Your treating team will be pleased that you are engaging actively and will support you in this process.

When it comes to choosing your medical team, it will be important to find healthcare professionals who have an interest in this area. This is covered in depth by Dr Heather King in the next chapter. There are now many doctors who take an active interest in lifestyle medicine and will be able to support the comprehensive changes you will be making. Even better if, like Heather and me, they have faced similar issues and are actively involved in improving their own health.

Making the space to recuperate

It is common that people with MS try and cling to their old lives and minimise the seriousness of the situation they are in. I remember telling the head of my department that I'd take a couple of weeks off and then come back to work. Fortunately, they demonstrated more insight than I did. MS is a major challenge to our physical and mental wellbeing. Our bodies have the capacity to heal and regenerate but we have to create the circumstances and choose the right nutrition for this to happen. This is a time to use the resources you have at your disposal to create the space to plan your recovery. Use sick leave entitlements, and claim on relevant insurance and income protection if you have them. Insurance companies are not always helpful in these circumstances and this is another time when having support around can be helpful.

It may be sensible to speak with your employer about the situation to see what adjustments are possible to make work life less demanding. These decisions are highly personal and dealt with in detail by people with MS who have themselves faced them in Chapters 14 and 15 on work and disclosure respectively.

The steps to recuperation and recovery

An important part of your recovery is engaging with the steps of the OMS Program. But, as we have seen, the support of friends and family is also critical. Make time to cultivate relationships. A good way to do this is to schedule regular times for relationship building. In this way we integrate the process into our lives and strengthen our connections. It can be particularly beneficial to choose activities that require thought and preparation. This will help improve the quality of our relationships, which is what really matters.

Make time to meet with friends and family on a regular basis, and cultivate relationships with people you care about

Social media can be a useful way of maintaining existing relationships and forging new ones. Take care to use it only as a 'way station'. If used to escape social interactions it can actually deepen a sense of loneliness and isolation.

On the following pages I briefly outline some ideas for getting started with the precepts of the OMS Program but this is dealt with in greater depth in the individual chapters of Part 2. In the early stages there are simple steps we can take that are enjoyable and move us forward.

Eating well is central to the OMS Program. This is a good time to explore new restaurants, particularly those that specialise in WFPB (wholefood plant-based) meals. Joining with friends on a plant-based cooking course is a good way to get started with the dietary changes. Many of the people involved in this area have overcome their own health difficulties and will be keen to share their knowledge with you. Their stories are inspiring and these interactions provide supportive social connectedness.

Nurture the mind–body connection. As mentioned earlier people are drawn to nature for healing and there is a lot of science that supports this. Being surrounded by nature has been shown to result in improvements in physical and mental health. Large studies have shown the positive effects of immersion in nature. It promotes the relaxation response and has beneficial effects on our physical and mental health. In many countries doctors can now prescribe time in nature. Other studies have demonstrated that even a simple view of nature can improve recovery after surgery. In Asia there is the long-standing evidence-based tradition of 'forest bathing'. 'Forest therapy' is now being adopted in the West.

'We should not exercise the body without the joint assistance of the mind; nor exercise the mind without the joint assistance of the body.'—Plato

Now is a great opportunity to explore mind–body practices like meditation, tai chi, yoga and the Wim Hof Method. The simple process of exploring these areas with like-minded people nurtures our social connectedness, further aiding our recovery.

Exercise is medicine and any exercise is beneficial in MS. It improves energy levels, cognition and mood, provides a neuro-regenerative effect, and has positive effects on the immune system, among many benefits. This is an opportunity to explore new activities and make new connections. If you are feeling more limited in your capabilities it may be helpful to speak with an exercise physiologist. They are well trained, highly knowledgeable and used to dealing with clients of varying levels of health and disability. They will be able to structure a program that suits you.

If possible, attend an OMS retreat, ideally with your partner or someone else close to you. This is a great way to kickstart your journey back to health. The retreats are run by people with expert knowledge of MS and the OMS Program. Many of the presenters have themselves recovered on the Program. They are an excellent opportunity to really get to grips with what is required and develop the mindset and skills to be well. Strong friendships often develop and these can provide a caring and nurturing support network going forward.

It is common at this time that relationships change. People whom we may not have felt so close to can come to occupy a much bigger part of our lives. Equally, some of those we feel closest to may become distant. Meditation and keeping our sense of purpose as we change our lives will help ease these transitions.

Further on down the road to good health

Being diagnosed with MS can be a gift. It can allow us to reconnect with our true self. The crisis point of an MS diagnosis is a wake-up call that we have been living a life out of balance. Many people with MS will recognise that they have been living a life that has not been serving them well. Keeping with our journey analogy, people with MS have been driving their car hard and neglected to take the measures required to keep it roadworthy. The first step is to pull over to the side of the road and get the emergency help required. As described above, this means taking some time out, accessing the healthcare we need—such as steroids for the immediate relapse—and then, if we wish to continue travelling in this vehicle (it's the only one we have), we are going to have to learn how to maintain it properly. Given what we know of the causes of MS, even if we hadn't developed MS, we were very likely to have gotten sick from another Western disease if we'd continued along that journey.

MS is an opportunity for people with MS to re-evaluate their lives, develop and grow. Most of us deep down have a sense of what we really want from life. Like many others who have faced serious illness, MS forced me to make the decisions that I had been avoiding. I needed help to get there. I needed the skills and knowledge of the OMS Program. Accessing meditation and psychology enabled me to achieve the peace of mind I required to act in ways to improve my health and make it happen. I also benefited from the support of a loving wife and family. My life is now much richer in so many ways and this would not have happened without MS or the OMS Program. Physically and mentally, I am in the best shape of my life—I feel better than I did in my twenties. It has transformed my view and practice of medicine. The OMS Program goes beyond helping those people with MS who find their way there and benefits their friends and families. Exit the road of sickness by following the sign marked OMS to a healthier and happier life.

Ground covered

The diagnosis of MS is a serious challenge to physical and mental wellbeing. It is crucial to express the grief and distress we feel so that we can move forward to make the changes required to successfully deal with this disease. The support of friends and family as we do this is invaluable. Take time out to recuperate from this time of ill health and make space to consider how life will need to change so that you can make the changes required to do well. The help of a psychologist and developing a meditation practice are useful in this process. Take medications if and when needed.

MS is largely due to lifestyle and environmental factors and its progression is nearly entirely due to these. For people with MS to do well, it is essential to adopt all the measures of the OMS Program as fully and as early as possible. Make your own decisions, develop the competence required to enact these choices and gather a supportive team around you to help. Nurture your relationships. Engage with your treating healthcare providers and take time to discuss your treatment options. There is an abundance of resources that will help you to develop the changes that you need to make. By combining the benefits of proven lifestyle interventions and medications, people with MS can expect to stabilise the disease and live happy and fulfilling lives relatively free of the burdens of MS and other Western diseases.

My Story:
Renee Coffey

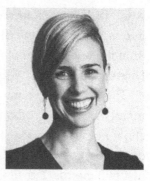

'You have two sizeable lesions on your spinal cord,' the neurologist said, pointing to two white smudges that looked no more sinister than any of the other surrounding white marks on my backlit MRI films. I was 29 years old and had just moved to Sydney, Australia, from my hometown in Brisbane to take up a significant promotion. I knew what those lesions meant, even if he wasn't saying it. I hadn't spent the last week obsessively Googling for nothing.

'There, there,' he said uneasily. 'Look, I could be telling you something really bad today. I could be telling you that you have advanced breast cancer.' I stared at him, mouth agape.

I wasn't told that day in 2011 that I had multiple sclerosis. I left his office with a scrap of paper saying 'transverse myelitis'; after I had insisted I got a reluctant verbal concession of 'probable multiple sclerosis'. 'What should I do now?' I pleaded as I was ushered out the door. 'Should I take some medication? Change my diet? Do anything different?' 'Nothing at all,' he replied. 'Just try not to think about it.' But that proved pretty difficult having just been told that I likely had a chronic, neurodegenerative disease with no known cure.

I recall those first two months after my diagnosis vividly. I remember entering a store, and finding myself looking through a stand of antique walking sticks to try and find the right one to buy to 'get it over with'. I remember receiving newsletters from a local MS society that advertised wheelchairs and shower aids; and I also remember the endless hours at night wondering whether I could ever have children or continue my career.

Then one afternoon, someone directed me to the OMS website. My cursor moved across the screen sceptically. What were they trying to sell me? With each click, my scepticism abated. Here was an evidence-based program developed by a professor of medicine, advocating for lifestyle modifications to improve the lives of people with MS. When Professor Jelinek's book arrived in the post, I read it in one 'sitting'—at the dinner table, in the bathtub and then in bed, until the early hours of the morning. And ever since that next day, I have followed the OMS Program and its recommendations.

The Program means so much to me. In the nine years since my initial diagnosis, I remain relapse-free. My latest MRI scans not only show no new disease activity, but one of the lesions on my spinal cord has completely disappeared and the other has shrunk to just millimetres. For the first time in my life I play and enjoy team sports—I am active, healthy and work hard to manage my stress levels, balancing a young family and a busy, continuing career.

Each year I celebrate my OMS-iversary with friends and family. And each year I am filled with gratitude for the journey that my MS diagnosis has taken me on and the role that the OMS Program has played in shaping this rich, rewarding life I get to live in good health.

11

Choosing your healthcare team

Dr Heather King

My life motto is to be happy, healthy and well—OMS
is the foundation.

Lenneke Keehan, London, UK, OMSer

A diagnosis of MS doesn't come with a map or even a GPS. One day you are well, then the next you may still be well but with the knowledge that there is a real possibility of a train wreck about to happen at any time. How to live with this uncertainty? How to find your path while engaging with life? It is not like one isn't already fully busy juggling commitments and carrying out plans each day. MS is like an unwelcome passenger forcing its way into the car that was already careering along and rather vocal in its demands for attention and pit stops.

It is now 28 years since my first episode, twenty since diagnosis and sixteen years since I accepted it. I can look back on the road travelled, and recollect the learning and the key people who helped me along the journey of life, a life that accommodated MS but was not controlled by it.

I was totally unaware of what lay ahead when the first episode happened, when I couldn't put the pegs on the washing line because my fingers mysteriously stopped working. My husband wisely said that 'a normal person would go to the doctor'. This episode resolved itself, and was diagnosed by the neurologist as 'mononeuritis, not likely to be MS as you have had no other symptoms'.

I was aware that I was stressed and busy with three young children and my work as a general practitioner (primary care physician). My dad bought me a dishwasher and life continued. I had my fourth child and life got even more hectic.

Eight years later, strange left-arm symptoms developed, so I went back to the doctor and the neurologist and had an MRI scan: the outcome was two lesions found and a referral to a neurologist specialising in MS. I was not prepared to accept the diagnosis, so named it in my head 'duo sclerosis', to be accepted as MS once I had four episodes, which was four years later. These days a prompt diagnosis gives an early start on modifying lifestyle and switching the disease off; but this was early days in my OMS journey and the lifestyle approach was certainly not on the radar of my neurologists.

At 61 I am relatively unscathed. On reflecting with my husband as I was preparing to write this chapter, we thought that perhaps our lives were even enriched by some of the choices we made because of that diagnosis so many years ago. Like a lot of life it all makes a lot more sense when you can review the paths taken, the choices made. The road taken becomes clear looking back.

Making significant lifestyle choices after a diagnosis of MS can actually enrich life; it has mine

I am a GP in a clinic that practises person-centred medicine where the needs of the patient, doctor and rest of the team are met. This has been of great help to me in figuring out my support team, which I have drawn from the medical and allied health professions, family, friends, work and the community.

A few years ago I was attending a self-management training course, run by Flinders University in South Australia, and I had a light bulb moment: *Oh my goodness, this is how it has been for me with my MS road trip.* The tools for self-management are exactly what I have developed from the team around me and from my learnings with the OMS Program. I have been blessed with very real support and autonomy.

The Flinders Program (www.flindersprogram.com.au) is described as a set of tools and processes that enable medical and health professionals to support their clients to more effectively self-manage their chronic conditions. The literature suggests that the following are important components of effective management of chronic disease:
- collaboration
- personalised care plans
- self-management education
- adherence to treatment
- follow-up and monitoring.

The research also suggests that programs that are successful in improving self-management have the following characteristics:
- targeting
- goal-setting
- planning.

Self-management support is aimed at helping the participant become an active, non-adversarial partner with healthcare providers.

But how do you get a team around you that you can work with? I started with my GP, chosen some years before, with whom I had a good relationship that had been built over time as I had babies, got treated for an episode of postnatal depression, and became overworked and tired. We had already covered some difficult ground, so I had trust in our ability to talk through situations, and his wisdom had been helpful in the past.

Then I had my fourth episode and was ready to listen. My GP told me an Australian medico, Professor George Jelinek, was speaking at an education meeting for doctors and he was attending because he had a patient who seemed to have 'switched his MS off' by following Jelinek's Program. Then my partner at work told me that she was going to pick me up and take me to hear what he had to say, something about controlling MS. To be invited to a meeting about 'your disease' is very confronting when one has been steadfastly practising denial.

Develop a plan

That meeting was life-changing. Prof Jelinek presented a detailed description of the cause of MS, of the immune system and of how to fight back. It was a watershed moment: here was someone who understood and was offering me a roadmap to take back control of my health and my life. The options were simple: sunshine, exercise, meditation and a diet low in saturated fat. Medication if required. To be offered a vision of escaping the vagaries of a disease that was totally unpredictable and disabling and be offered hope and a plan of action was so empowering. It seemed like I could resume planning my life again.

I made a visit to discuss my options with the GP. He was very supportive, noting the dietary and lifestyle benefits of the Program and that it certainly would reduce my chance of developing the type 2 diabetes and obesity that run in my family. Then he shared that actually he was vegetarian and meditated himself, and that philosophy and mindfulness had been of great benefit to him.

Build your team

Step 1: Choosing a good GP

It is very important that you have a doctor you can talk to, who listens, supports your goals for wellness, and encourages compliance with the OMS Program. It may be that you already have a GP who can fill this need, but you may need to talk to them and make the connection around your OMS recovery plan. Perhaps they know that MS can be moderated and even prevented, perhaps they don't. Educate them, lend them the *Overcoming Multiple Sclerosis* book, show them the OMS website.

Choosing your healthcare team starts with finding a good, understanding general practitioner (primary care physician)

Being a doctor-patient with a dreaded disease that is incurable is heart-sinking. A patient who is taking control and saying, 'Look I've got this plan, can you help and support me?' is exciting and gives the doctor something to work with. So much of the doctor's day-to-day role is encouraging lifestyle changes, often with little patient buy-in or success. It is uplifting to have someone who is actually positively working on their diet, mindfulness, meditation and exercise. Prescribing some vitamin D is a small thing and can be a pleasure.

With the GP on board with your program, if episodes or health issues crop up, they are already engaged. They are likely to help you to access the resources you need to meet your goals of wellness.

Step 2: Finding a neurologist

With diagnosis comes the need to engage a neurologist, the specialist who can organise MRI scans and apply for the specialised MS drugs. Neurologists are conservatively trained and may be less supportive of holistic lifestyle changes. Some will be downright discouraging; others are on board with the OMS philosophy. When I was feeling a bit unsupported, as if it was only the 'disease' that was being looked at, a neurologist from a different field said I had to figure out what were the right questions to ask my neurologist. He told me that my neurologist was never going to be able to answer the 'touchy-feely' questions and advised me to find someone else for those questions. It's so crucial to find a neurologist who is not going to undermine you.

On a day-to-day basis, the neurologist may not be as involved in your care plan as you may have expected. Often they will provide an overview of your medical condition, monitor progress and determine the very specialised disease-modifying medications that are available. And of course, in many places in the world, they can figure out the various funding requirements. They may have access to and knowledge of appropriate physiotherapists, rehabilitation programs and gyms where MS is understood and well managed. If you have a relapse then you really need your specialist. Their wisdom and expertise are vital. Feeling supported, being able to trust their advice on when to scan, when to use high-dose steroids and when to involve powerful immune suppressant drugs is invaluable.

Step 3: Accessing allied health

In New Zealand, where I live, there is usually an MS nurse available through the health system. This is the person who may well provide more general support, have an ear to the ground for the OMS Program and give advice about available support systems. They may also smooth medication supply issues and follow up on specialist authority drug applications. If you seem to be hitting a roadblock, the MS nurse often has a way to sort it out for you. They know 'what is out there'.

A lot of the difficulty with MS is either fearing what may happen or being frightened when episodes do happen. In my experience, many with the condition find it hard to face the fact that there is a problem and that one has a vulnerable nervous system at all. There is a risk of losing one's way and the emotional rollercoaster can certainly take its toll.

There are many allied health resources available for people with MS

Very early in my journey I decided to see a psychologist to see whether any of the angst and stressors of my life were triggering my immune system in a way that resulted in neurological inflammation. The immune system works in mysterious ways and I was ready to try anything. It is also one of the recommendations in the OMS Program.

The psychologist had a particular interest in the mind–body connection and we spent a few years on and off working on my concerns. It was fascinating and life-changing. The personal growth I experienced was gradual and my relationship with my husband was able to accommodate the ructions along the way. We look back now and see how beneficial it has been to both of us and how fortunate we were to have a health trigger that forced me to spend the time and money to seek psychological help and endure the associated discomfort. I regard it as one of my most life-enriching experiences.

MS can affect any part of the body, but as all these parts can be troublesome in one health setting or another, there are services for everything. A person who is largely well in themselves but has a specific issue such as an isolated bladder disturbance is someone who may well benefit from specialist expertise.

If I think about my medical history, there have been many specialist and allied health professionals involved, not all for MS, but most systems have been covered! Postnatal referral to the bladder physiotherapist was valuable for their expertise in stress incontinence, a problem that affects many women, with MS or without. They have skills that are also useful for men, which they make available through hospital urology units or continence services. I have had referrals to physiotherapists with special interest in neurological conditions who were very supportive after an episode affecting my leg strength. Having a therapist who does a comprehensive examination and then advises on what you can do to improve is very supportive and shows a way forward. Word of mouth helped me find a funded rehabilitation gym to use for some months.

A friend sent me to a physiotherapist she knew who recommended a particular splint and Nordic poles, the poles used for cross-country skiing, for my mild foot drop. I could then trek New Zealand's Queen Charlotte Sounds Great Walk (a very good trek if you are not too confident in your ability as there is a boat to carry your heavy gear and you can get a ride to the next point if it is too arduous or you need a day off; I skipped the big hill but otherwise had a ball doing the track with my family). Doing some training walks with a specialist Nordic walking trainer on correct technique was amazing. I was back to walking at speed, with balance and purpose. She told me that I could walk forever as long as I kept up my technique. I repeated these words to myself as I slogged up hills and towards the end of the longer days on the Great Walk. I have cherished my walking poles (Black Diamond carbon fibre Z poles that fold into my knapsack and go anywhere a walk might be in the offing).

The foot drop was affecting my horse riding so I did some research and the occupational therapist at the Riding for the Disabled Association suggested a stirrup wedge that kept the foot straight even as it tired. People have been so kind when looking for a solution for me.

I found an orthopaedic surgeon brave enough to look into my foot drop, which never fitted in with the pattern of my MS episodes and, as it turns out, it was actually spinal stenosis, not MS, and his surgery has tremendously improved it. It is worth continuing to search for answers, even if it means looking outside the specialty of neurology.

An osteopath with magic hands soothed aching parts of my body and eased headaches and seemed to have a healing presence. She healed my soul in times of stress. A respiratory physiotherapist was able to help with disordered breathing that I first noticed in antenatal classes; perhaps you know that desperate need to gasp and breathe as soon as the instructor starts doing the relaxing breathing part of the program? I am so glad that I have put the effort into learning diaphragmatic breathing. It has made meditation and sleep so much easier. I have gone back for a few extra visits when overstressed and the upper chest breathing pattern recurs. As soon as I notice a couple of deep sighs, I am onto it: resetting the breathing, practising a moment of mindfulness and breathing out.

Finding professionals who will support you with MS but also look to tending to the rest of your health is critical, remembering that we age in all aspects of our body and MS does not exclude other conditions. Know yourself and your body. 'Does this feel usual for you or different?' This can be important, and something that you can then discuss with your doctor. Being listened to and being heard, being validated, will bolster your morale. It may not happen with every encounter or with every health practitioner but it is vital that we all have some relationships in our lives where we are being heard and being asked how we are feeling.

We may not think of family, friends, neighbours and work-mates as part of our health team, but they are the ones who have heard others' stories and experiences, what has worked for someone else. You may find you get unsolicited and unhelpful advice along the path but don't be deterred by it; you can test

Friends and family can form part of your healthcare network

the ideas with a more medically minded friend or your GP or MS nurse.

Learn as much as you can and teach those around you

Your family, friends, neighbours and workmates are the ones that know you best and have the energy to encourage you forward. They may be able to identify the multiple cobwebs that hold you back with the inertia of change avoidance. Get them on board as part of your team, show them your vision and if you can be clear about what direction you are taking, they will be behind you as your support team, offering a helping hand or a word of encouragement.

My workplace added salmon to the shared lunch shopping list and changed to a dairy-free spread. We already had salad vegetables and fruit at work, so minimal change was required. There are many possibilities.

When my close friends (the small playgroup we had set up for our children) heard about the retreat for people with MS at the Gawler Foundation in Australia, they decreed that I was going and they would come to Melbourne with me to send me off in style. Before I knew it, airfares were booked, a delightful boutique hotel in Melbourne was reserved for a couple of nights, a bed and breakfast in the mountains and lunch in the Yarra Valley were organised, all to be enjoyed with my friends before I was to be delivered to the retreat centre. My concerns about the four children and finances were brushed aside; they said that I could not afford *not* to do it as taking control of MS was a pivotal decision not only for me, but for my family and husband, too. If I could remain well it would be life-changing for everyone. And so it has proven.

I was terrified of joining this group of people with MS. In the past I had undertaken sessions with the psychologist over my fears around accepting the diagnosis of MS. I felt like a wild kitten being put in a cage, legs and claws out-stretched, all fluff and teeth. With the kind encouragement of all involved in the retreat, I was able to move through the fear to a point of acceptance. Not to say that I wasn't filled with trepidation as we got to the mountains the night before and it was tears all round as they dropped me off.

Meeting the other participants was surprisingly a solace rather than a trauma. These were people who understood what weird tingling or unexpected weakness felt like and the whole life disarray that this condition was causing, not only with the immediate symptoms but the uncertainty it created for one's future. Then there was the retreat itself. I absorbed every teaching: the education around MS, the tools around medication and self-care, forgiveness and storytelling, the dietary advice, the science behind each of the OMS interventions. Here was a whole toolkit in one place.

Keep in touch with yourself physically, emotionally and spiritually

Taking time for myself in such a beautiful setting meant that I could reflect on my life, sit and ponder, 'what is the question I need to answer today?'. Taking time to perform some forgiveness rituals, letting go of various hurts and traumas, was invaluable. Here I learned the value of being me. That only I can live my life and this is not selfish, but essential. If I am not for me, who is? If I am only for me, what then? Finding a community that understands and validates these concerns is very empowering and enabling.

I look to my life now and appreciate the balance that is vital to my day-to-day health: the joy and energy that I feel as I handle and ride my horse, the solace of stroking the cat and the well-being that I enjoy as I sit on the rug looking into the fire with a cup of tea on a cold winter's night. The beauty and truth of the natural world are what centre me and bring me to wholeness. In truth my support is more than the medical profession, more than therapists, more even than friends and community: it comes from moments of beauty and connection in nature and the recentring of myself each day.

When I had my first baby, a sister-in-law said, 'You will get loads of well-meaning advice, just choose to follow the ideas that suit you.' Perhaps this is true in every aspect of our lives. It certainly helps to have a well-researched guide like the OMS Program as many aspects of it have been reviewed and interrogated. When initially diagnosed I was surprised at how many well-intentioned alternative suggestions were made to me, presented as 'facts' and 'definitely' effective no matter how way-out. Following a middle ground is always a challenge, and choosing a support team that you trust and are well grounded is a great solace. If you have to have MS with you on life's journey, let's choose some great travel companions to help spread the load.

In summary, get support to understand MS as a disease, how it's affecting you and what is required of you to manage it, then build a team of medical and non-medical people to help you along the way. This sets you up to self-manage and head into life with joy and confidence.

Overall, I would stress the features of the Flinders Program in your self-management. Be someone who:

- has knowledge of your condition
- follows a treatment plan (care plan) agreed with your medical and health professionals
- actively shares in decision-making with your medical and health professionals
- monitors and manages signs and symptoms of your condition
- manages the impact of the condition on your physical, emotional and social life
- adopts a lifestyle that promotes health
- has confidence, access to and the ability to use support services.

I wish you a safe and enriching journey; in life it is the travel that is important whatever the destination.

Kia hora te marino, Kia whakapapa pounamu te moana, kia tere te Kārohirohi I mua I tōu huarahi.

May the calm be widespread, may the ocean glisten as greenstone, may the shimmer of light ever dance across your pathway.

My Story: Caroline Clarke

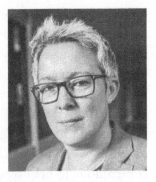

I was diagnosed with something called transverse myelitis (spinal cord inflammation) back in 2007. I was semiparalysed for a few weeks, and took about a year to recover with the help of lots of great physical therapy, and then thought little of it (I assumed that I'd had a 'weird neurological incident'), until I received a classic 'MS hug' (strong discomfort around my chest) about eight years later. I happened to be the chief finance officer of a hospital, so I was able to consult and get an MS diagnosis relatively speedily from my colleagues—in hindsight I think that was very lucky, although it must have been very strange for them to have to deliver the news to a colleague. Consequently, I decided to take my treatment to another hospital, not because I lacked faith in their services—far from it—but because I wanted to separate my day job from the serious business of overcoming MS. I later became CEO of the same hospital group, and I still think it was the right decision—I'm totally open about my diagnosis but I'm there to lead the organisation, not to be a patient.

I live and work in London, which is blessed with many large specialist teaching hospitals, and tons of great neurological teams, doing masses of research. I was very keen to get to a team that had lots of patients like me—mid-forties, with active relapsing remitting disease, that might benefit from some of the newer treatments. And so I was given two rounds of alemtuzumab infusions over the course of 2016 and 2017. Taking a holistic approach to managing my condition was also really important, so, like many people newly diagnosed, I scanned the internet for advice on how to help myself, and whether there was anything I could do to control my symptoms through lifestyle adjustments. After an initial strange experimental period with organ meat and other unusual programs, I discovered Prof Jelinek's *Overcoming Multiple Sclerosis* book and began to follow the OMS Program. It made total sense to me and was only going to improve my life.

Coincidentally, a colleague at work introduced me to Linda and Tony Bloom, who literally live a mile away from my main hospital. So it was super easy to engage with OMS and learn more about the team and the organisation, and to be motivated to promote the Program to people newly diagnosed with MS. I wish that I had been directed to the Program earlier on, and that I hadn't gone on my strange dietary journey to find it.

I'm really glad that my initial diagnosis was accompanied by an optimistic outlook from all the neurologists I saw—I think that was helpful in how I framed the condition. And having a team that understands that you can contribute massively to your own health outcome is also important—we are not passive as patients, and having encouragement from medical and health professionals to investigate what's out there, and to support life-style changes as a way of halting disease progression and aiding recovery, is key.

12

Mental health

Dr Keryn Taylor

My recovery from MS (yes, I said 'recovery') is way ahead of expectations; I've regained enough balance to stop using a cane, I have noticeably less fatigue, I've regained cognitive skills.

Tom Jones, St Petersburg, USA, OMSer

Mental illness, particularly depression, is a common problem for people with MS. In fact, about half of all people with MS will experience depression. Depression can have a big impact on day-to-day life and also affect physical health. Although people with MS need to be aware that they are susceptible to mental health problems, this knowledge can leave them feeling worried about their future. But what is equally important to know is that there is much that can be done to take care of one's mental health, in terms of prevention and also treatment of symptoms.

A healthy lifestyle is not only excellent for the physical health of those with MS, it's also great for their mental health. The OMS Program has all bases covered, from reducing the risk of becoming depressed to facilitating recovery from depression and other mental health problems. Outside of the Program, there are many strategies to support mental health, including talking to a healthcare professional, engaging in creative therapies, building strong social connections and taking medication if needed.

Feeling stressed? Anxious? Or depressed?

When first diagnosed with MS you might experience a range of emotions. You could feel shocked and be incredulous that this is really happening. Symptoms of MS can be so varied and take years to develop, so you might have spent some time worrying about what was wrong with your body before being diagnosed, or been uncertain about whether symptoms were caused by MS or another serious illness.

Once diagnosed, people often feel anxious about lots of issues relating to their diagnosis and how it will impact their health, family and future. It is completely understandable to feel sad or angry about a diagnosis of MS and current or anticipated losses. Such feelings should not be seen as not coping or a sign that you are becoming mentally unwell. It is important to express your emotions with people who care about you. These experiences are covered in detail in Chapter 10, 'I've just been diagnosed with MS'.

Experiencing a range of emotions in response to MS is normal and does not necessarily mean you are becoming anxious, depressed, or otherwise mentally unwell

How do I know if I am becoming anxious or depressed?

After a diagnosis of MS, or during any challenging time in life, difficult emotions may start to dominate life. If you start to notice that you are feeling worried or very stressed a lot of the time, or sad or tearful, it's important to recognise this could be the start of a more serious problem such as anxiety or depression that needs attention. Particularly if these emotions occur on most days, for more than a week or two. Sometimes you might not notice the signs yourself, but others who care about you may notice the changes and be concerned.

Is anxiety becoming a problem for me?

It is understandable to feel anxious about MS. This is a natural human response given the fear and uncertainty that MS can generate, especially about having a relapse or becoming disabled. From an evolutionary perspective, feeling worried can in fact be helpful as it focuses attention and can be a motivating force for change. But if anxiety starts to arise a lot of the time and affects day-to-day life, it's important to recognise that it has become a problem. Anxiety can be a different experience for different people. Some people might feel like they just can't relax and are on edge and feel tightness in their body. Others might not be sleeping well and feel tired and grumpy. Some people might notice that any physical symptom can lead to panic about a relapse even if another cause is much more likely.

These symptoms that might not have bothered you before you were diagnosed with MS might keep you feeling 'on high alert' and for some can cause intense feelings of fear and worry. As Associate Professor Craig Hassed describes in Chapter 6, the long-term toll of stress, anxiety and depression can have a major effect on our physical health and can lead to serious physical and mental illness. It's important to recognise the early warning signs of feeling stressed or becoming anxious or depressed and take active steps to prevent them becoming a problem.

Am I becoming depressed?

You may notice feelings of sadness, or feel easily irritated or that you no longer enjoy things the way you used to. There may be changes in appetite or weight. These might be symptoms of depression. People who are experiencing depression often have trouble sleeping: either sleeping too much or not being able to get to sleep or maintain it. Trouble sleeping is often accompanied by feeling tired and low in energy. People can feel slow in their body and in their thinking and find it

Look out for the early signs of anxiety and depression and talk with someone you trust

hard to concentrate. Sometimes people feel overwhelmed by MS and start to feel that life is not worthwhile. It is always important to speak with someone you trust if you think you might be depressed: it might be a friend, family member or a healthcare professional.

How depression affects people with MS

Mental illness, particularly depression, is a common, under-diagnosed and under-treated problem for people with MS. Depression is the single-most important factor that can affect day-to-day life, even more so than disability or fatigue.

We know that depression is more common for people with MS than for people with other chronic illnesses. There is something very specific about MS that increases the chances of depression, not just the impact of adjusting to having a serious illness. Overall, approximately half of all people with MS will experience depression at some point during the illness. If you are experiencing these symptoms, it is important to know that you are not alone.

Mental illness is also a very common problem for everyone, with or without MS. In the general population one in four people will be diagnosed with a mental illness during their life, with mood disorders like anxiety and depression being the most common. So, some people diagnosed with MS may already have experienced anxiety, depression or an episode of another mental illness. This does not necessarily mean that MS is going to cause an episode of depression again, but you may be more vulnerable and it is particularly important to look after your mental health and seek support early if difficulties arise. If you have previously had serious challenges with mental illness, it is especially important to surround yourself with a strong medical team to support your mental and physical health.

Depression is a common medical illness, affecting around half of all people with MS at some time during the illness

How depression affects MS itself

We know that an unhealthy lifestyle combined with the stress of diagnosis and adjusting to MS can lead to high levels of stress hormones and inflammation. We also know that inflammation is a common pathway in MS, depression and other mental illness. Having MS and becoming depressed may lead to greater inflammation and a worsening of the physical illness, which can then lead to a worsening depression, setting up a vicious cycle. However, there are many ways to stop this cycle and to turn it around, particularly strategies that reduce inflammation and optimise immune function. Feeling better physically makes you feel better mentally and vice versa, so preventing and managing depression are key in managing overall health and MS.

Depression and MS both increase inflammation in our bodies, with the inflammation from untreated depression driving further MS activity

Will changing my lifestyle improve my mental health?

Making healthy choices about diet, exercise, mindfulness and stress-reduction strategies, not smoking, and drinking alcohol in moderation are important for both physical and mental health. In healthcare, lifestyle modification is an evidence-based secondary and tertiary preventive medical approach, often called 'lifestyle medicine'. This area of medicine involves the benefits that a healthy lifestyle can bring both physically and mentally and has the added psychological benefit of providing patients with personal control over their health and future.

The OMS Program is a great example of evidence-based lifestyle medicine and what can be done to improve physical and mental health for people with MS. Preventing a further physical relapse through lifestyle modification may be an obvious goal for a person with relapsing remitting MS. 'Relapse prevention' is also a commonly used concept in mental health, and describes what can be done to prevent further episodes of mental illness.

Changing or optimising lifestyle is a hugely effective aspect of preventive medicine, capable of preventing both the onset of depression and recurrence of episodes of depression or other mental illness.

All parts of the OMS Program can benefit mental health and improve resilience. We know that for people with MS, having an ultra-healthy diet, taking omega-3 supplements and undertaking exercise and meditation are all helpful in combating depression, as is vitamin D, which can help prevent, and reduce the risk of, depression while improving cognitive function.

Choosing to modify and maintain a healthy lifestyle is the foundation for good mental health; all steps of the OMS Program benefit mental health

Can diet and supplements improve my mental health?

For all of us the saying is true: if you eat well, you feel well. A plant-based wholefood diet plus seafood, with no meat or dairy, as described in this book, is the optimal diet for good general health and wellbeing. Not surprisingly, it also brings benefits specifically for mental health, and for people with MS who follow the OMS diet, the risk of depression is reduced. Furthermore, supplementing with a plant-based omega-3 like flaxseed oil, as recommended in this book, offers many health benefits including reducing the risk of depression. Supplementing with vitamin D as recommended by the OMS Program is also associated with a lower risk of depression for people with MS.

When eating a varied plant-based wholefood diet there is generally no need to take any further supplements for your mental health. If depression or anxiety are a problem, it is a good idea to ask your GP (primary care

Eating well and supplementing with flaxseed oil and vitamin D reduce the risk of depression and are likely to improve overall mental health

physician) to check your iron levels; a deficiency generally only occurs occasionally for women of child-bearing age, but can be easily treated by iron supplements. Please also make sure that the GP checks your thyroid function and vitamin D and vitamin B12 levels.

Exercise, fatigue and sleep

There are so many benefits to being as physically active as possible. Exercise releases feel-good hormones, including endorphins, into the body, has a positive effect on mood and the immune system, and reduces inflammation. Not surprisingly, regular exercise is associated with a lower risk of depression for people with MS. The more people exercise, regardless of the level of disability, the lower the risk of depression and the better overall mental health. More great news about exercise is that it is one of the only evidence-based interventions shown to improve fatigue for people with MS. We know that fatigue is a symptom of both MS and depression, and if people experience fatigue they are more likely to experience depression. Regular exercise can act as a 'circuit breaker' between fatigue and depression, providing huge benefits for people with MS.

So to sum up, exercise can directly improve fatigue symptoms but also reduces the risk of depression, improves cognitive function and improves overall mental wellbeing.

Getting a good night's sleep

If you think you might be anxious or depressed, a good question to ask yourself is 'how well am I sleeping?' The answer can provide a good indication of overall mental health. In fact, sleep has been described as the mental health equivalent of temperature for physical health. Sleep really is essential for good health, but it can also be easily disrupted. Sleep difficulties can also start if there are physical symptoms of MS such as pain or incontinence, and a cycle can occur where physical symptoms cause poor sleep, which has a negative impact on mood, leading to further difficulties sleeping. Focusing on ways to improve sleep can often turn this around. Most people need 7–8 hours of sleep each night. It is helpful to know how much sleep you need and to aim to regularly achieve this amount.

Basic strategies like keeping a regular bedtime and wake-up time are extremely important. Being active and not sleeping during the day will help to improve your quality of sleep. Creating a habit of getting outside during the day, especially in the morning into sunlight and enjoying the outdoors and nature has dual benefits for circadian rhythm and mood. While napping and resting during the day can seem like a good idea, this can actually reduce your ability to sleep well at night. If you do really need to nap during the day, try to limit the time to less than twenty minutes.

The final essential step for good sleep is to have a regular routine at bedtime that helps in winding down, including reducing stimulus like screen time and TV during the hour before sleep and keeping the sleep environment cool and dark. A mindful approach to sleeping is extremely helpful: on nights when it is hard to sleep be kind to yourself and non-judgemental. As one's meditation and mindfulness practice develop, sleep and energy improve.

Please see your doctor to help with relief of any physical symptoms that impact on sleep. It is best to avoid sleeping tablets as these can cause more problems for sleep in the long term.

Staying as physically active as possible and making sleep a top priority will reduce fatigue and have benefits for your mental health

The impact of alcohol on mental health

Drinking alcohol can be a social and enjoyable part of life for some people and in general there is no medical reason why people with MS should avoid drinking alcohol completely. Drinking alcohol in moderation has been associated with a number of good mental health outcomes for people with MS, including a lower risk of depression and a greater chance of recovering from depression. Some people will choose not to drink alcohol and of course that is okay.

Alcohol affects people to different degrees but generally makes people feel initially more relaxed. However, the later effects of alcohol are not as positive and people can feel more anxious or depressed the day after. If you think anxiety or depression are becoming a problem, it is wise to either avoid or limit alcohol intake. Alcohol also interrupts the quality of sleep, which can then have a negative impact on mental health.

It is clear that drinking alcohol heavily is likely to lead to worse health outcomes for people with or without MS. If alcohol has become a problem for you, it is important that you take steps to address your drinking first. Reducing intake or stopping completely usually results in feeling better physically and mentally and sleep will improve as well. Going alcohol-free for a month is worth a try to see if any benefits are noticeable.

Alcohol in moderation may be beneficial for some people's mental health, while for others avoiding or limiting alcohol is the best choice; being a non-smoker benefits both physical and mental health

Not smoking is one of the most important things that people with MS can do for their physical health. Being a non-smoker is also beneficial for mental health and is associated with a lower chance of depression over time for people with MS. It is thought that the neurotoxic effects of and immune changes due to cigarette smoking are harmful for both MS and depression. The importance of stopping smoking has been emphasised throughout this book.

Talking to a healthcare professional

For anyone diagnosed with a serious physical illness such as MS, having someone to share your feelings with, help you to adjust and cope with challenges and encourage you to build on strengths can be a stabilising force in the journey to overcoming MS and staying well. Many people will have someone to turn to, whether that is a partner, family member or friend, and those people play a hugely important role. But there is something very different about talking with a healthcare professional: this experience can provide an opportunity to talk about your biggest fears about MS without worrying about burdening the listener and also allows objective feedback and strategies for improving aspects of health and life.

There are a range of clinicians and types of therapies that can be helpful. The best clinician to first speak with is your GP, who will be able to recommend someone best suited to your needs. That could be a counsellor, psychologist or psychotherapist. Clinicians will have different backgrounds and it is worth asking your GP to recommend someone with experience helping people with MS and lifestyle medicine or mindfulness. Another important consideration in your choice of clinician is the connection and ease that you feel with those you consult. Hopefully, this will happen with the first clinician you meet, but if it doesn't, keep trying until you meet someone who you feel you can talk to and who really listens. Your GP might recommend that you see a psychiatrist, who will be able to provide psychological strategies or talking therapies and also provide medication if required.

The most common and evidence-based types of talking therapies for people with MS are mindfulness-based therapies and cognitive behavioural therapy. There are a range of other therapies that can be helpful and most clinicians will have experience in a range of techniques. In Chapter 6 Associate Professor Craig Hassed provides an excellent overview of mindfulness-based interventions, including meditation, which has immense benefits for our mental health.

Talking with a healthcare professional is a valuable opportunity to explore emotions around MS and to build strategies to improve and maintain mental health

An important part of strong mental health is to have a good understanding of who you are. All of us are born with different temperaments and develop different personalities. Early in life we build patterns of thinking and relating to others that continue across our life. These patterns are often enduring and have a habit of repeating themselves. Talking with a health-care professional can help you to identify any unhelpful patterns and make new choices and create healthier ways of thinking and relating, both with others, but also with ourselves.

We all have strengths and vulnerabilities in how we relate to others and in how we think about life and view the world. A diagnosis of MS is life-changing and is an opportunity to reflect on who you are, what is important to you and what you want for your future.

A useful starting point is to ask yourself: *How have I managed past stressful times in my life? What were things that helped and what were things that didn't work out so well?* I have a diagnosis of MS: *What strengths can I use and what areas can I improve and build on? Who are the people in my life that I can count on and who are the people who often leave me feeling worse about myself or my situation?*

Another good question is: *How would someone who knows me well describe me?* You might be known in your family as 'a worrier', which you might think is completely unhelpful with a diagnosis of MS, particularly if you worry excessively. But this trait can also mean that you are very good at paying attention to detail and seeking out information, a big positive after a diagnosis of a serious illness like MS. Even aspects of ourselves that might be seen as vulnerabilities can be managed, reframed and used as strengths.

Talking to a healthcare professional can help you to understand how a diagnosis of MS has affected your life and assist you to build strengths and understand vulnerabilities

Engaging with a clinician to help improve your mental health is a worthwhile undertaking that people often find benefits them more than they expect. But for many it is not an accessible option. Other good strategies include using writing, music or art to express emotions.

Simply writing down thoughts and feelings about MS can be very helpful and has even been linked to better immune function and fewer health problems over time. The exercise of finding a quiet space and writing whatever comes to mind about the diagnosis of MS, then reflecting on the writing and any feelings that arise can be a beneficial exercise. You might find that you write about frustrations or losses relating to MS but also things that you are thankful for. It can be worth writing about what strengths and supports you have and what goals you want to work towards.

Writing regularly in a journal can be particularly helpful as it allows the opportunity to look back and see how you managed to get through challenges, providing motivation for the present. You might find that you identify times during the day, week or even year where challenges occur more often or life seems harder. You can channel this information into thinking about strategies to help navigate these difficulties. In the next chapter on building resilience, Dr Rachael Hunter outlines more of the benefits of writing and making time for pleasure and purpose in life.

Music and art therapy are creative modalities that can bring many benefits to overall health and can help an individual to process difficult emotions and experiences. We know that music can strongly influence how we feel, so making choices about what we listen to on a regular basis can be really helpful for our mental wellbeing. You can easily access free online resources; for example, if you enter 'music, images and relaxation' you will find videos with images accompanied by music, which can add to the experience. Music therapy is an evidence-based intervention that has been shown to improve quality of life, motivation and mood for people with MS. Music therapy may involve listening to, playing or even writing music or lyrics. Art therapy can involve any medium; people might paint dark pictures of difficult times or colourful scenes reflecting hope. Art has been shown to improve self-efficacy and mental health in people with MS. What's more, there is no need to have any previous experience in art or music for them to benefit your mental health. You can search online by entering 'music' or 'art' and 'association' to see whether there are therapists available in the local area.

Other strategies include visualisation, such as visualising nerve cells being repaired and covered in myelin, and guided imagery. A clinician can help you use the latter to enter into a state of relaxation and engage in visualisation, which might involve imagining yourself in a place where you feel positive about your health and future with MS.

Writing, music and art are excellent and healthy ways to express emotions

Whether you enjoy writing, music, art or imagery, there are many creative modalities you can engage with to look after your mental health. The next chapter on resilience provides more strategies to proactively maintain and improve your mental health.

Staying socially connected

It is said that a problem shared is a problem halved and it is important for all of us to have people who care about us and who will be there during both the good and darker days. For people with MS there is a strong relationship between having people from whom you can seek support and a lower risk of depression. All relationships take time and effort and a diagnosis of MS can quickly bring changes to many relationships. Some relationships will strengthen and others that you thought you could count on may no longer be there for you. To become and stay well it is vital to invest wisely in relationships that support you and your health. In Chapter 9 on families, Drs Sandra Neate and Pia Jelinek discuss relationships with partners and how they can positively influence mental health within the context of the OMS Program.

A good way to connect with others who understand what it is like to be diagnosed with MS is to connect with the OMS community. At first people might feel overwhelmed by the idea of talking with others who have MS. They might not want others to know about their diagnosis of MS and desire to keep it private. People might worry that others will treat them differently, feel sorry for them or discriminate against them. These fears can become a burden and weigh them down, leading to less social connection and a greater chance of becoming depressed.

The OMS charity offers a number of excellent supports that help foster connection with others. These resources provide valuable emotional support, given they link people to other positive and proactive members of the OMS community. People with MS who are engaged with the OMS Program certainly have better mental health. Research examining the benefit of the OMS Program found that people who read *Overcoming Multiple Sclerosis*, visited the OMS website or attended an OMS retreat had a much lower chance of depression, less fatigue and significantly better quality of life.

Engaging with the OMS community in any way is good for your mental health but the more you engage, the better you feel. People who had no contact with the Program had ten times the risk of depression. The benefits are both immediate and long-lasting; for instance, we know that people who have attended OMS retreats have improved quality of life and better mental health five years after attending a retreat. This is a remarkable result given that the outlook for people with MS and their mental health is typically so poor.

Building strong social connections will help to support mental health; there are many benefits to linking in with the OMS community and resources

You can find more information about these OMS supports at www.overcomingms.org or by contacting the OMS charity's head office in the United Kingdom. There are also many other MS organisations and support groups with helpful resources.

Dr Rachael Hunter further discusses the importance of lifestyle and connection in the next chapter, 'Building resilience'.

Medication

The first step in preventing and recovering from anxiety and depression is to optimise or make changes to lifestyle. Psychological strategies are the next step in addressing or preventing problems with mental health. If difficulties continue and symptoms for a person with MS reach a point where it is hard for them to do day-to-day activities, then more help is needed. Medication can play an important role in recovery from a serious episode of anxiety, depression or other mental illness.

The most commonly prescribed medications for depression are a group of medications called selective serotonin reuptake inhibitors or SSRIs. This type of medication tends to have fewer side effects than other antidepressants. For most people with MS other types of antidepressant medications such as tricyclic antidepressants are not a good choice because of their effect on bladder function and sedating effects. Yet for some, these drugs can be helpful for sleep and pain relief. The choice of antidepressant is best made by considering the potential side effects of the medication and how these might positively or negatively impact on any MS symptoms.

As with all decisions relating to medication, it is a good idea to research the options and decide for yourself which choice will give the most benefit with the least chance of side effects. Of course, you need to discuss the options with your doctor before starting medication. Antidepressant medications are taken each day and are most effective when taken for at least one year, but do not have to be taken forever.

Antidepressant medication can improve mental health for people with significant depression

It is not good practice to treat anxiety, depression or any mental illness with medication only. People with MS who are anxious or depressed and require medication have a greater chance of recovering if they also maintain a healthy lifestyle, engage in psychological therapy and maintain strong social connections.

Some medications prescribed for MS can affect mental health. Interferon can cause depression and even short courses of steroids can cause sleep disruption and changes to mood. If you have concerns about any MS medications, always speak to your GP or neurologist.

Partners' mental health

In Chapter 9 on families, Drs Neate and Jelinek emphasise that the mental health of a person with MS has a huge influence on their partner's quality of life. It is therefore important for the person with MS to look after their mental health for their own benefit, but also to benefit their partner. The mental health of partners and other people who support a person with MS can be affected in both positive and negative ways by MS. Partners of people with MS may also experience stress, anxiety and depression as they navigate challenges that MS can bring.

Partners need to be aware of signs that they are under stress and to take action if they develop symptoms of anxiety or depression. And they should remember that if they make healthy lifestyle changes and actively engage in managing stress, they are likely to enjoy better mental health. For some people, seeking help together as a couple can be a good way forward if difficulties arise in the relationship.

It is important for both people with MS and their partners to actively look after their mental health

The process of working together to find solutions, with the help of a clinician, can be a therapeutic process with enduring benefits for all.

Ground covered

A diagnosis of MS elicits a range of emotions and it is important to recognise the early signs of significant anxiety or depression. Although depression is very common for people with MS, there is a lot we can do to prevent it from occurring or help to recover from it. To overcome MS and live well, it is important to invest time and energy looking after our mental health. A healthy lifestyle as described in this book is the foundation for good mental and physical health. Other important ways to improve mental health include talking to a healthcare professional, engaging in creative therapies and actively building strong social connections, including with other people with MS. Medication can be a further building block in recovering from serious episodes of depression or other mental illness.

My Story: Fran Barclay

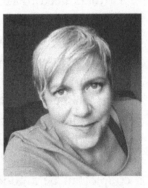

I wasn't climbing mountains, swimming oceans or running marathons before MS. Life was filled with children, friends, laughter, work, dancing and other domestic 'adventures'. MS brought that all to a halt when I collapsed two days after reluctantly agreeing to my estranged husband moving in with me after he lost yet another job and with it his accommodation. Our son was eight and our daughter only eleven months old. After twenty years of rocky union and then separation, our children and I once again felt somewhat trapped and dependent in an extremely difficult situation.

Given this ongoing stress, it was perhaps no surprise that I began to develop a variety of symptoms. My neck was painfully tight, my extremities aching and cold, vision blurry, legs non-responsive and crippling fatigue never left me. There followed various medical tests seeking an explanation.

Wheeled into an appointment with my neurologist, I was looking for answers, but more importantly, hope. I got half of what I sought. Finally locating my file, he bluntly diagnosed MS and recommended 'massive doses of IV steroids with a one in two possibility of *losing* [my] hip joints'. This dismissive, red-faced man had already written me off, regarding my body parts as expendable.

With the diagnosis came a frightening shrinking not only of my brain but of the world around me and my place within it. What followed was eighteen months of painful, bedridden guilt and self-loathing. Unable to undertake daily mothering tasks or even pick up my baby, I felt worthless and afraid. Hope was barely there, reduced to just a dim and flickering kernel.

When able, I devoured as much information as I could, from mainstream portents of doom to the downright bizarre and everywhere in between. My quest stoked the awakening phoenix within me. I was not giving up. External hope finally came in the pages of Professor George Jelinek's book *Overcoming Multiple Sclerosis*. I could see my goals and started making incremental steps towards achieving them.

Through the global OMS community I have met the most remarkable, resilient individuals who have inspired me to hope. With them I have shared the setbacks, failures and triumphs of living with this disease, and provided and received support through shared understanding, experience and commitment. I came to recognise and appreciate my own inner strength—the me who knew I had a future beyond what that particular neurologist saw all those years earlier.

I love and am loved, and cherish my lifelong friendships. My life overflows with love and daily gratitude. My children are now 22 and 14. I hope they will learn that while physical health can support mental health, physical health without resilient mental health is nothing. My goals were to lift my inner girl again and to dance in the embrace of a beloved. I still don't climb mountains, swim oceans or run marathons but I have achieved both of my ambitions and more besides. How blessed I am to have a spirit that refuses to be broken! I remain the mistress of my own fate.

13

Building resilience

Dr Rachael Hunter

> OMS is to me a revelation, an education, an inspiration and a shining light of positivity, hope, support and warmth.
>
> *Richard Burt, London, UK, OMSer*

If there truly was a formula for developing resilience everyone would want to buy it. People would seek to avoid the challenges and traumas of life if they could, wouldn't they? But ironically, if we avoided all those challenges, all the failures and frustrations, we would learn nothing. We would not grow. We would be less than we have the potential to be. Because it is through the challenges and the heartbreak that people are forced to dig deep inside themselves to keep going. To rebuild themselves when they feel broken. To keep going when they may want to give up. And in doing so they may find a strength that they did not know they had. They may create a life that they did not even know they wanted. People can find hope in the darkest of places. And so, if there were a formula for sale that helped you avoid all of that, would you honestly buy it?

What is resilience?

It seems that resilience does not mean a life without challenges or adversities—in fact, the road to resilience may be characterised by more than its fair share of struggles. What is more, a resilient person doesn't deny or minimise challenges, nor do they pretend that things are not tough. In fact, a resilient person is just as likely, if not *more* likely, to notice when they need help, acknowledge that things are tough and reach out to others. A resilient person recognises that finding things difficult or struggling is not a sign of weakness, or something to be ashamed of. Sometimes things really are just hard.

While resilience is often described as the ability to 'bounce back' after setbacks and challenges, and this certainly may be true, in reality resilience is about much more than being able to get back to 'normal'. Firstly, getting back to how things were may simply not be possible; secondly, you may not *want* to return to your previous situation. In contrast, true resilience may be described as the capacity to keep going *despite* those setbacks. To accept the challenges that may lie ahead. To be changed by the experience but not defeated. Like the gnarly tree on the side of the hill, whose roots stand fast but whose branches have had to curve with the wind in order to survive, you may bend but not break.

For many people a traumatic event can shatter their assumptions about themselves and the world, triggering a new appreciation of life and a humbling awareness of personal vulnerability. By coping and adapting, a new sense of identity may emerge.

Historically, researchers have focused on understanding trauma and emotional distress rather than resilience. This focus makes sense, because being tuned into dangers has kept us safe. But by focusing too much on the negative effects of challenge and trauma, other valuable lessons about coping and resilience may be missed. The truth is that many people survive so many different traumas and challenges all over the world, every day. Many of those people have faced devastating traumas and instead of being defined or broken by them, they somehow emerge stronger, more compassionate and hopeful. What defines those people is not just that they refuse to give up, but they also somehow *shift* in response to the experience. This adaptation and the ability to keep going are regarded as resilience. And so, by studying those people, we have begun to develop clearer understandings about what resilience looks like.

Resilience may be described as the ability to adapt in response to challenges

It can be helpful to think of resilience as a muscle—the more you exercise it, the more familiar and stronger it will become. In the same way cooking often helps you to be a better cook, or practising yoga can help flexibility. Regularly exercising the behaviours associated with resilience can help it become a more natural and instinctive response. Over time it will start to become part of who you are. Research has shown a wide range of actions and behaviours to be associated with resilience and well-being, and the good news is that these are largely ordinary actions and behaviours available to everyone. It can be helpful to think of them as falling into three categories that are easy to remember as the three Ps: *Pleasure, Purpose and Practice.*

Are your basic needs being met?

Before exploring those three important Ps, it's important to be sure that *basic*, physical needs are being met. If those needs aren't being met adequately, building resilience is going to be much more difficult. In the same way that you might check over your car before a long journey, ensuring that the engine has oil and water, you need to regularly check in with yourself. For example, are you making sure you are hydrated? Are you getting regular and enough sleep? Do you feel safe in your home? Some people find it helpful to check in regularly in a journal and keep track of how these aspects of their life are going. Take some time now to think about your life and your 'building blocks'. The framework in Figure 13.1 may be a helpful guide.

Once you have considered these underlying building blocks, you can turn your attention to how you can build resilience in your day-to-day life. Research has helped to establish a good understanding of the characteristics of resilience: *taking control, hope, connection to community, a sense of personal agency or control, optimism and adaptability,* to name just a few. In many ways adopting the OMS Program gives a head start on this. But sometimes it can be

How to build resilience

Food	OMS
Avoid sugar highs, or 'hunger' lows Steer clear of vegan 'junk' food* Avoid emotional eating	Plant-based wholefood diet Regular exercise Stress management Vitamin D3 and omega-3 Medication if necessary

Sleep	Hydration	Security
Follow regular sleep routine Reduce caffeine intake Optimise room temperature	Drink enough water	Financial security Safety Love

Figure 13.1: The 'building blocks' of resilience. *Note: not all vegan food is healthy; it can be processed and high in sugar and bad fats.

hard to think about how to make the changes associated with resilience. This is where the three Ps may be useful—see Figure 13.2. The framework offers a simple way to develop your own personal plan or 'prescription' for building resilience.

Pleasure

A life-changing diagnosis can cause people to re-evaluate life and ask themselves, *what truly makes me happy?* It can bring into focus what is most important to them, how they want to spend their time and with whom. Arguably, the harder things are in life, the more important it is to experience a sense of pleasure and joy. But far from being a cliché, there is now a growing body of evidence that experiencing pleasure and positive emotions is a really simple and effective way to help build a person's psychological resources—in other words, to help people to cope with stress and challenges.

The protective effects of integrating more pleasure into life occur in part because when people spend time *doing* things they enjoy, these things not only make them feel good at an emotional

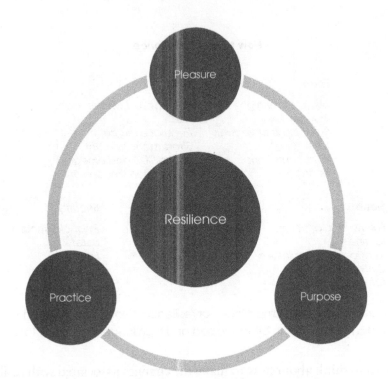

Figure 13.2: The 3 Ps framework for building resilience.
Source: R. A. Hunter, 'Clinician and Service User's Perspective on Managing MS: Pleasure, Purpose, Practice', *Front Psychol.* 2020;11: 709.

level but also contribute to the production of important neuro-chemicals including oxytocin—sometimes called the 'pleasure hormone'. Oxytocin has positive physical and psychological effects and enhances feelings of confidence, making people more sociable and strengthening relationships. It can help to improve mood and provide a sense of optimism, which will help one to manage stress more effectively. It makes sense, doesn't it? We all know that when we are feeling happy or more positive it can be easier to cope with the 'bumps in the road', right?

After receiving a diagnosis like MS and living with the sense of uncertainty it can present, it is understandable that at times it may feel that life is hard. While incorporating more pleasure into day-to-day life may seem an obvious and all too easy place to start, some people can find it tricky. Many people find it difficult to put themselves first, and many people look after other's needs before their own. It may take a lot of hard work to allow more joy and pleasure into life, and it may be best to start by believing that you deserve it. A good way to get a feel for this is to start by recognising that prioritising pleasure and joy is essential for physical as well as emotional health—see it as part of the prescription for wellness.

Protective effects of experiencing pleasure and joy are both psychological and physiological; however, we may need to work to find pleasure and overcome a natural instinct to look for negatives

Try keeping a list of pleasurable moments that you notice throughout the day—these may be sensory, social or emotional. It may be the satisfaction of finishing a crossword, or the taste of some freshly brewed coffee. It may be the shared joy of laughing with friends, or the feeling of peace experienced when in nature. By the end of the day it may be a surprise to find how much is on the list.

A good way to increase the amount of pleasure in each day is to be quite practical about it. Perhaps even write a diary (see Table 13.1) simple things that could be included in the day that give pleasure or a sense of contentment. There may be times of the day or week that are more challenging, and these can be especially useful times to plan something enjoyable. Everyone's life is different, and the things that give us pleasure will also be different. The key is to find what's pleasurable and meaningful to you and integrate more of it into your day and week. This kind of structured approach suits many people. Others of course may find that a more free-form style of writing in their journal when it feels right in whatever format feels best suits them better. Remember, the OMS Program is all about choices. Choose whatever format suits you best.

Recording these things in a diary may seem like too simple a task to be meaningful, but acknowledging that you deserve to feel pleasure, and considering ways in which you can incorporate this into your daily routine, can be a big deal for many people.

Table 13.1: Diary of daily 'pleasures'

	Mon	Tues	Wed	Thurs	Fri	Sat	Sun
morning	Walk with a friend						Walk to buy a newspaper
afternoon	Rest	Swim		Bake biscuits	Rest		
evening			Book club			Watch a movie	

Once you notice and integrate more pleasure into life you will find it easier to pause and pay attention to those moments. You will start to look forward to them and find that they also bring unexpected benefits. For example, taking a daily walk to buy the newspaper that you enjoy reading will also connect you socially— with the shopkeeper who you might get to know, and the people you pass on the street. It will help you to get outside in the fresh air and have some gentle exercise.

Paying attention to these pleasurable moments connects us to the present and builds a more mindful way of being in the world. We often fall into the trap of spending too much time worrying about the past and a future that hasn't even happened yet. As human beings we have evolved to look for the negatives—in fact, this has served an important evolutionary purpose and helped to keep us safe. But while worry can be protective, it can also be hard to shut our minds off from these worries. People's lives today are filled with distractions and you may feel like you have a lot to be worried or thinking about. But becoming caught up in these worries and distractions too much can trigger all sorts of unhelpful feelings and this can be problematic in the long term. By cultivating a more mindful way of being in the world you can get less caught up in your thoughts or worries. In Chapter 6, Professor Hassed provides an excellent overview of the benefits of mindfulness and describes ways to introduce this practice into day-to-day life.

If your attention is drawn back to worry or sadness, that's okay. It would be unrealistic to say that life is all about pleasure and joy—it's not. In fact, some people may have to deal with more uncertainty or pain than others, especially when living with a chronic condition. But by working towards *accepting* that pain or uncertainty, through self-compassion or mindfulness for example, we avoid our attention becoming focused on it, or getting caught up in it. By disengaging with that frustration or 'fight', we are free to notice and enjoy life's pleasures. In fact, for people who may feel like they have very little control, this is one powerful means of creating some control—over where and how they focus their attention. Even in some of life's most difficult situations, there are always opportunities to experience simple pleasures.

> *By accepting uncertainty we can disengage from 'fighting' MS and free ourselves up to notice life's pleasures*

Purpose

When embarking on an important journey, it is likely that you know the purpose of the trip, where you are going, *and why*. Likewise, purpose is an essential component of a fulfilling and happy life. But life can get very busy and people become so caught up in the 'what' and 'how' of life that they forget about the 'why'. Receiving a life-changing diagnosis like MS can be a big wake-up call and trigger a lot of soul-searching about what is truly meaningful. The diagnosis of and living with MS can provide an unexpected opportunity to explore and connect with your true values and sense of purpose. This can be really helpful and has also been shown to be very protective, increasing wellbeing and reducing symptoms of depression. As the revered neurologist Viktor Frankl wrote in his account on his experiences in the Nazi concentration camps of World War II, 'those who have a "why" to live, can bear with almost any "how"'.

A sense of purpose and meaning can be derived from belonging to, or serving, something bigger than oneself. This may be most simply understood as something like a religion or social cause, but could just as easily be related to something less spiritual—like the local community, creative expression/arts or a person's role within the family. What all of these examples point to is a sense of belonging and community with essential opportunities for authenticity, contribution and connection to others. Some find this when they join the OMS community, on the website forum or in OMS Circles around the world.

For some people a sense of purpose may be obvious, but this is not true for everyone. Some people find it helpful to talk about it to close friends and family—you will be surprised by how much other people value these conversations and how they can strengthen your relationships. If you feel a bit overwhelmed, there's a simple exercise used in various forms in acceptance and commitment therapy that can be used to help clarify values. It's a way of exploring what you would like to treat as important in life, and beginning to think about how to work towards that. I like to frame it in the following way:

> Imagine it is your 80th birthday party. At this party, people who are important to you, and to whom you are important, have come together to celebrate you and your life. When the time comes at this party for people to make speeches about you, they will spend their time talking about the kind of person they experienced you to be. What you stood for. How you affected their life. Take some time to consider this and don't limit yourself to what your mind currently tells you is achievable; you're simply exploring a possible direction for your life.
>
> When you have finished the exercise bring your mind back to the here and now. Use the questions below to help you reflect:
> - What did you identify as important to you?
> - What was it like to consider what you stand for?
> - What emerged as important in your life, values and accomplishments?
> - What might you do in the short, medium and long term to help this become a reality?

Understanding more about our values can help us to create a life that is more in tune with our purpose and values. This can present more opportunities for experiencing connection with others, moments of pleasure and a sense of fulfilment. Connection to community and purpose is also a great source of comfort, direction and support when times are hard, providing opportunities to support others in a meaningful way too. Remarkably, a sense of purpose has also been associated with a range of health benefits including reduced cognitive decline and a strengthened immune system.

Take some time to think about your purpose and values. What gives life meaning? How might you contribute to the world? What is your 'why'?

Being mindful of our purpose and values may also provide valuable insight into situations or relationships in our life that no longer align with those values. This may help you to identify situations that may be contributing to chronic stress, or that you no longer feel supported by or connected to. You may begin to ask yourself: *Does this situation help me or drain me?* With growing awareness and self-compassion, you may feel able to move away from any unhelpful situations and commit to prioritising your own wellbeing.

Practice

People who demonstrate resilience and healthy emotional wellbeing don't have a superpower, but one thing they all do is practise the behaviours associated with resilience consistently. In particular, they practise what we might understand as simple, regular acts of self-care. When we talk about self-care, we often think of health spas or soaking in a hot tub. And while this may be part of it, good self-care could be any number of behaviours or actions that nourish emotional, physical and spiritual wellbeing. Importantly, it is the regularity and repetition of these small but important acts of self-care that make them so powerful.

Creating new routines for exercise and physical activity is one example. Exercise is essential for maintaining positive mental health and remaining active plays a key role in the OMS Program. Finding what works for you is the key—some people like to exercise on their own while others prefer being part of a group or exercising with friends. However you like to do it, creating a regular practice or routine helps many people to maintain the benefits.

Doing activities outside has the added benefits of helping you spend time in nature or in the fresh air, both of which have their own health benefits, not to mention the added bonus of getting vitamin D. Being active with other people can also provide a wonderful sense of community as well as the encouragement that you may sometimes need to keep going (or to get going!). Working towards a 'goal' can help provide a focus and a great sense of accomplishment when you manage to finally achieve it. In Chapter 5, Dr Stuart White discusses the value of exercise and a range of ways in which people can regularly engage in physical activity.

Developing methods to manage stress and encourage a more mindful outlook not only contributes to resilience but is an important part of the OMS Program. In particular, the benefits of meditation and mindfulness are well established. Even so, some people can find it hard to develop and maintain a regular practice so remember that it is very common to find it challenging to begin with. You might find it helpful to use an app to get started, or guided meditations. Or you might like to really throw yourself into it and sign up to a course online or in a group setting—this can be a great way to begin as you will get lots of support and encouragement.

Some people find that it suits them more to introduce 'mini-meditations' or 'mindful moments' throughout their day. You can find details about meditation and mindfulness in Chapter 6. However you approach it, remember that many people find it easiest to start small and build gradually. Another really good way to build a practice is to attach it to an activity that you already routinely do. This is the most effective way to start and sustain this kind of practice. For example, taking care to be truly present when walking could make a daily walk a walking meditation. Or, if you always boil the kettle for some morning tea, you could practise a breathing exercise or 'mini-meditation' while you wait for it to boil. Or take a 'mindful moment' to think about a gratitude list while brushing your teeth before bed. Creating these simple, daily practices by linking them with an established routine can help to build the practice—and moving forward this can contribute to a positive feeling of accomplishment.

There are a number of other ways to practise healthy stress management. For example, in addition to what has been discussed above, there are many other benefits to journaling—keeping a written log or 'diary' of feelings, thoughts or worries. There is now a good body of evidence to show the benefits of writing—these include not only emotional benefits and reduced rates of trauma, but also physical benefits such as protective effects for the immune system. As well, journaling can provide a helpful record of events and symptoms—it can be very rewarding to look back over time and see how much things have improved or changed. If you enjoy more creative ways of expression, such as through art or music, this may be what you choose to help manage stress. Whatever you choose, creating a regular practice for reflection or emotional expression to help manage stress can bring many benefits.

Importantly, by recognising the value of these regular self-care behaviours, you are creating an acknowledgment that you are worthy of care. This may feel quite difficult at first, but accepting yourself and your situation with kindness can be truly healing. Consider how you would talk to a friend who was in your situation and seeking your advice. What would you say? How would you talk to them? Practising talking to yourself in the same way will cultivate self-compassion and kindness for yourself, as well as empathy for others. To truly accept yourself with compassion and kindness you may also need to let go of regrets, old resentments or situations in your life that simply cannot be changed. Holding on to them may only be contributing to feelings of stress. And while it may be hard, compassion, and in some cases

There are many different types of self-care, behaviours and actions that contribute to resilience—they may be physical, emotional or even spiritual

forgiveness, can help the process of letting go of difficult feelings that you may be holding on to. Finding a way to let go of these situations (if possible) can be truly freeing and allow you to accept yourself and your situation more freely. Paradoxically, in the spirit of change that often accompanies adoption of the OMS Program, a diagnosis of MS can be a good excuse for addressing some of these long-held difficulties.

So practising self-care can take many different forms. And creating practices that support wellbeing can have a range of benefits. Those practices may be physical, emotional or even spiritual. What is clear is that setting the intention and committing to some or all of these practices can help to build resilience and contribute to wellness.

A personal approach to resilience

Every individual is unique, and every person will have their own unique experience of MS. Take some time to develop your own personal approach to building resilience. You can use the three Ps to help or you may just want to develop your own ideas. What's important is to remember that building resilience doesn't have to be complicated; in fact, the behaviours and habits of resilient people are available to us all.

While a diagnosis of MS can be life-changing, there are very few people who have an easy journey in life, with or without MS. In reality, there are very likely to be more bumps in the road ahead for us all. But resilience can emerge from challenging situations and by adapting to those challenges and developing behaviours that bring us pleasure and align with our purpose, with practice difficult roads can lead to beautiful destinations.

Ground covered

There are many ways in which we can build resilience in our lives and the OMS Program gives us a good head start. Being diagnosed and living with MS can be challenging, but resilience often emerges from the most challenging situations. When living with MS, it is important to take control of the things we can do in our day-to-day lives to build resilience and maintain our emotional and physical wellbeing. Resilience is associated with a whole range of thoughts, actions and behaviours—all of which are available to everyone. Responding to the challenges with flexibility and self-compassion is important. Daily practices and behaviours that bring pleasure to our lives, and that align with our values, have all been shown to contribute to resilience.

My Story: Dr Saray Stancic

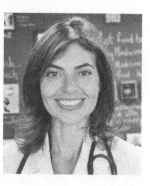

After four gruelling years of medical school and two years of an internal medicine residency, I could finally breathe a sigh of relief as I entered the third and final year of the residency. This year, I was sure, would be largely a breeze compared to what I had just endured. The second year of residency had been by far the worst: countless sleepless nights at the hospital, stressful morning rounds, evenings at home studying for yet another exam. I understood the sacrifices needed to achieve my dream to become a physician. I was willing to endure them. But what came next seemed cruel and unfair.

It happened abruptly. In between tending to patient care issues I had found time to take a nap during a busy overnight shift at the hospital. About thirty minutes into sleep, a nurse paged me to evaluate a patient in the ER. When I tried to get up my legs were completely numb. I could see they were still there but could feel nothing. Fear swept over me. After hours in the radiology suite undergoing MRI scans of my brain and spinal cord, I first heard the dreadful news: 'You have MS'.

This wasn't supposed to happen; it felt like the end before I had even begun. I was now a patient with an incurable chronic degenerative disease. I was told that I should prepare to be disabled within twenty years.

I resolved to do anything to slow this disease. I fully entrusted the advice that my expert physicians would offer and followed all recommendations, remaining compliant with their treatment plan. But even though I followed their counsel, within a few years I grew dependent on multiple medications and increasingly weaker. About eight years after the diagnosis, I was dependent on a cane and largely demoralised and depressed.

Then, by chance, I came across an article written by Dr Roy Swank describing his hypothesis on diet and its influence on MS. This opened a door—the door that changed my life. It was in that moment that I began to search the literature, putting together the puzzle pieces that would lead to a comprehensive understanding, empowering me to introduce sweeping lifestyle changes into my life. I learned about the importance of a plant-centred, fibre-rich diet, the value of daily movement, the value of addressing streams of stress and discovering how to sleep effectively, free of prescriptive 'crutches'.

It was undoubtedly these simple changes that altered the course of my life from suffering and dependency on a cane, to joy and crossing the finish line at a marathon. In 2020, medication free, I commemorated 25 years of living with MS with a 25-mile walk. The lesson was to cease resisting and accept what life had placed in my path, all while trusting that it was the experience I needed to have in order to arrive at my purpose. It may seem cliché, but it is so very true: *what doesn't break us does indeed make us stronger*. To me, resilience is the ability to persevere, even in the face of seemingly unrelenting adversity. So, thank you MS for the challenges, pain and loss you presented me— you have made me resilient beyond measure.

14

Work

Rebecca Hoover

The OMS Program has made me feel empowered that I can change the course of this disease and do not have to accept an inevitable decline into disability.

Jo Watson, Perth, Australia, OMSer

Why re-envisioning work with MS is often necessary

Being diagnosed with MS is almost always frightening and often leads to the person reconsidering what to do about their work and career. Many may be surprised to learn that even though MS may necessitate significant career changes, it probably won't. In fact, for many an MS diagnosis puts them on a road to achievement not previously seen as possible. Instead of setting low expectations, aim high!

In the past, working with MS was often viewed as an almost insurmountable challenge because so few people with MS were knowledgeable about the lifestyle programs that can actually change the course of MS and improve outcomes. If you have been exposed to this 'insurmountability' narrative, consider a few people who have lived with MS.

Senator Paul Wellstone from Minnesota served in the United States (US) Senate despite having MS and considered running for president. Another interesting US political leader is Bill Bradbury from Oregon who, after being diagnosed with MS, went on to serve as a legislator, as the president of the state senate in Oregon and, for many years, as the Oregon Secretary of State. Or consider world-renowned author Joan Didion, who was diagnosed with MS in her late thirties; she went on to write award-winning fiction and non-fiction works and is now in her eighties. Along the way she was nominated and became a finalist for a Pulitzer Prize for a book written in her sixties. Obviously, MS did not stand in the way of these individuals. They have set examples that help us to re-envision what is possible for those with MS. People with MS are found in almost all types of careers throughout the world, many of them very demanding, as illustrated by most of this book's chapter authors and other contributors.

It is also true that MS does not usually cut careers short. Consider my own career. I turned 70 last year and currently work as an information technology and financial manager. In my sixties I realised that I would be able to work past age 70 if I wanted to and could delay receiving social security benefits until age 70. The US Social Security program provides pensions for older US citizens, with the largest benefits going to the less than 4 per cent of recipients who delay receiving benefits until age 70. As a person with MS, being able to delay receipt of social security benefits until age 70 has given me a real boost and inspired a lot of other people with MS. Clearly MS does not have to be a barrier.

In the past, MS was seen as an almost insurmountable barrier to continuing in work, but not any more

As information about the relationship between lifestyle choices and MS outcomes becomes more widely available, an increasing number of people with MS are living long, productive and vibrant lives. Indeed, only about 5 per cent of those with MS are likely to have unavoidable severe disability with MS. When thinking about work, it is important to remind ourselves that most of us are able to overcome many MS symptoms with lifestyle changes involving diet, the use of a few supplements, exercise, stress reduction, and so on. Some may find drugs helpful.

It is also important to remind ourselves that many formidable career and work plans are achievable by people with MS. At the same time, we need to be realistic because there may be many hazards along that road. Individuals with MS who plan to have careers need to know about the hazards and how to overcome them.

It is worth our time to learn approaches to addressing work-related issues because people with MS work for many reasons, including economic, psychological and social benefits. Those with MS who continue to work report higher quality of life than those who do not work. Psychological problems are less common in people with MS who work than in those who do not work. While sometimes hard to believe, work is often fun and can improve lives.

Working with MS often requires a detailed map

There are many issues that might arise for a person working with MS; the physical problems caused by MS are only some of the issues to be addressed. Working with MS not only involves managing MS as a disease, it also involves securing good job matches and addressing potential discrimination and psychological issues. Figure 14.1 illustrates the many problems that may arise when with working with MS, together with suggested solutions.

In management sciences the situation with work and MS is recognised as complicated to the extent that what is called an unstructured problem-formulation and decision-making approach is often recommended (an 'unstructured' approach is one that is used when even the definition of a problem is difficult to tie down and where a broad view of issues works best). Figure 14.1 is a problem-formulation diagram and shows how comprehensive and complicated the situation with MS and work can become. It lists groups of problems related to MS and work on the left and appropriate solutions on the right. So, for example, the first problem involving the timing of decisions is matched with a solution involving improved timing as a result of improved knowledge of MS. Sorting the potential problems into categories and identifying solutions by problem category makes the matter of mastering work when we have MS much easier.

While there are many problems that might arise for a person with MS who continues to work, there are also many solutions

Figure 14.1 shows five types of problems that may arise working with MS: poor decision timing, poor job matches, psychological issues, discrimination, and physical limitations caused by MS. It is also important to consider that following the OMS Program is a critical step on the road to maximising the chances of a long and successful career. As discussed in the following pages, the OMS principles can help with the psychological problems that often occur with MS, with the social problem of discrimination and with the physical problems that MS can cause.

In the remainder of this section, we will discuss the problems as outlined in Figure 14.1 and their corresponding solutions.

Untimely decisions

Some of the biggest mistakes made by people with MS involve making premature decisions shortly after they receive the diagnosis. Imagine driving down a road and a sinkhole opens up and swallows both you and your vehicle. An MS diagnosis can feel like that career-wise. Many instinctively believe that career and work goals and dreams must be abandoned so all efforts can be devoted to merely surviving the MS sinkhole. Realistically, this is usually an overreaction. By far the most frequent work-related hazard comes not from the diagnosis of MS itself but from an overreaction to the MS diagnosis. It is important to realise that most people have less to fear than they imagine.

Consider again my own experience. I was diagnosed when little was known about the importance of lifestyle changes in overcoming MS and I floundered along still working but not doing all that well because of physical difficulties. Once a year, I experienced a nasty relapse that definitely caused work-related problems. I imagined my life heading downhill fast. After about eight years with the disease, I learned of Professor Roy Swank's diet for MS and happened to start taking vitamin D3 supplements

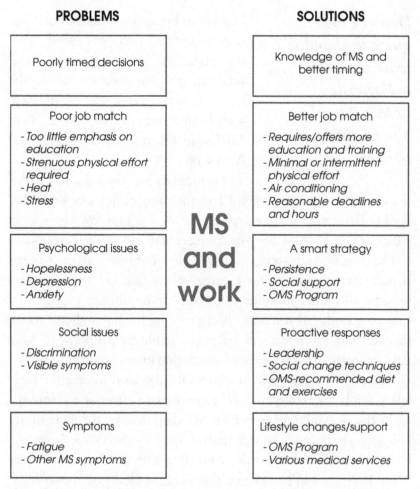

PROBLEMS	SOLUTIONS
Poorly timed decisions	Knowledge of MS and better timing
Poor job match - *Too little emphasis on education* - *Strenuous physical effort required* - *Heat* - *Stress*	Better job match - *Requires/offers more education and training* - *Minimal or intermittent physical effort* - *Air conditioning* - *Reasonable deadlines and hours*
Psychological issues - *Hopelessness* - *Depression* - *Anxiety*	A smart strategy - *Persistence* - *Social support* - *OMS Program*
Social issues - *Discrimination* - *Visible symptoms*	Proactive responses - *Leadership* - *Social change techniques* - *OMS-recommended diet and exercises*
Symptoms - *Fatigue* - *Other MS symptoms*	Lifestyle changes/support - *OMS Program* - *Various medical services*

MS and work

Figure 14.1: Types of problems encountered by people with MS at work and suggested solutions

for pre-osteoporosis. Changing my diet based on Professor Swank's recommendations and adding vitamin D3 supplements changed my life. I had one relatively mild relapse and then no more relapses after that. I was diagnosed with MS about 30 years ago but I have gone two decades without a relapse. I still have minor symptoms that are not visible to others but MS has not affected my career since I made the necessary lifestyle changes.

Since first learning about the importance of lifestyle changes, I became familiar with the OMS Program and have found that

Don't be too quick to abandon work soon after a diagnosis of MS; this is almost always an overreaction

I feel even better as a result of making improvements recommended in the Program. My MRI scans have reflected this improvement also. My lesion volume was lower on my last scan than it was initially on my first MRI scan taken about 30 years ago. Amazing!

Fortunately for me, I did not make drastic career changes when I had the early difficulties with MS. Rather than making career plans during the first few years with MS, it is best to make lifestyle changes first and allow their potential healing impacts to play out and then consider career changes if necessary. Or if you have career plans that are important to you, by all means continue to pursue them with the expectation that your health, if you make lifestyle changes, may well not stand in your way. Most careers are very doable by people with MS. And remember that if you are considering major changes to work, or indeed stopping work, re-entry into the workforce after time away can be more difficult and require extra effort and planning.

In the beginning of either an MS diagnosis or the start of an MS lifestyle improvement initiative such as the OMS Program, a sensible approach is to take your time with making major decisions. If things don't work out, there will be plenty of opportunity later to address issues as they arise.

Poor job matches

There is relatively little research about which factors contribute to or detract from successful work experiences for those with MS. In the limited research available, a few variables are mentioned relatively frequently. These range from the nature of the job to psychological issues and discrimination.

Research shows that some jobs are better suited to people with MS, especially when they are experiencing some common symptoms or some level of disability. The jobs that researchers find most likely to suit people with MS have a few factors in common. These are: high educational level, work not requiring a lot of physical strength or sustained physical effort, comfortable working temperatures and not undue stress.

People with MS who hold jobs requiring higher levels of education earn more and have longer and more satisfying careers but note that this factor involves the opportunity for control. When given a choice, many people with MS undertake further education or training. Savvy individuals with MS understand that education can translate to increased wages and job satisfaction. If you have an opportunity to pursue more education, it is usually advisable to do so.

Consider jobs that fit better with MS-related issues that people with MS might face

The role of educational level works for individuals with MS just as it works for those without MS. As a general rule, those with the most education earn the highest salaries. Avoiding jobs requiring physical strength and sustained physical effort may be necessary in some instances. If you have substantial physical disabilities, it is probably not realistic to pursue a career as a professional football or basketball player with MS. Likewise, jobs in trades that involve sustained physical exertion for hours may prove difficult. However, many with MS work as physicians, nurses and other health professionals, and in other jobs requiring greater use of brain than brawn.

Typically the best work environments for people with MS have comfortable temperatures. Heat is an important factor for many with MS. Because heat can cause fatigue and a perceived worsening of symptoms, working in comfortable conditions is usually wise.

Many with MS feel that high-stress jobs contribute to MS relapses or problems and that stress is a factor that detracts from employment success, while others find that work stress and pressure are powerful motivators and bring out the best in them. Stress, however, can be mitigated for many people with the help of meditation or social support. It does make sense to try mitigating stress before making other decisions that would result in reduced income.

It is frequently noted that the process of improving one's life-style helps individuals develop a sense of self-control and better enables them to defer gratification. There are psychological and social benefits from this. It is interesting that scientists find that the ability to defer gratification is a factor that predicts both high levels of income and wealth accumulation. Experts recommend that everyone, with or without diseases such as MS, learn to defer gratification. Yes, indeed, developing the habits needed to follow the OMS Program may help to make you prosperous.

Psychological issues

Almost everyone with an MS diagnosis experiences feelings of hopelessness, anxiety and depression in the early stages. These emotions are common and quite normal and do not mean that you are mentally ill. Rather they reflect you are going through a difficult time. Learning to manage the entirely normal psycho-logical issues associated with an MS diagnosis can help you to stay on top career-wise. You can take control of your own psycho-logical wellbeing. The research shows that people with MS who do the best resolve early to be persistent and to overcome MS to the extent that is possible for them.

Persistence is a major factor in work-related success and one can resolve to be persistent. The importance of this factor in long-term career success for those with MS is great news. Each person has complete control over the amount of persistence they display.

It helps to have a sense of humour about the failures that one can encounter early in a career. If you don't have failures, you are not trying very hard. Learn to laugh about the mistakes you make when trying to launch your career. Mistakes keep us humble.

Research again and again finds that social support can help us through almost any situation. One idea involves finding an MS mentor. Many older individuals have had MS for decades and have learned a great deal about how to manage the disease and navigate difficult work situations. It is smart to find MS mentors who can provide ideas and moral support. Look for such individ-uals in MS groups, online support groups or even among friends and acquaintances. It's best to avoid those who claim to have miraculous MS treatments or who want to charge for mentorship. Someone who acts as a mentor to others but constantly tries to sell books or services is not a true mentor.

You are best off looking for someone who is happy to help without expecting anything in return.

Social support and mentorship can be very valuable in maintaining employment

It is important to know that following the OMS Program can help with psychological issues. Eating the plant-based wholefood diet recommended by the Program is key not only for physical reasons but for psychological reasons as well. Using the Program to ensure good nourishment is wise and well described by Dr Keryn Taylor in Chapter 12 on mental health. Likewise, the exercise recommended helps to prevent and alleviate anxiety and depression. The Program tends to be the basis for most other steps needed to help improve employment-related outcomes.

Social issues: discrimination

Despite the career success of many people with MS, the problem of discrimination remains and it happens a lot more than it should. Research shows that people with MS often earn lower wages and have lower rates of workforce participation than those without MS. One factor that is often key in prompting discrimination is the visibility of MS symptoms. Another contributing factor is gender, since women often earn less than men in substantially equivalent positions. Women with MS can therefore be victims of discrimination based on both gender and disability.

Men with MS, unfortunately, also seem to encounter employment-related discrimination. Men with MS are actually less likely than women with MS to work. The withdrawal of men with MS from the workforce has not been studied. However, since men often have jobs in the trades and perform work that requires physical exertion, it may be that some men with MS are less able to cope with the physical demands of work.

For both men and women, discrimination is not uncommon, and a plan for mitigating the impact of discrimination or seeking legal assistance may be needed. There are many strategies for addressing discrimination.

Proactively addressing discrimination

Researchers suggest there are two ways to address discrimination: emotion-centred methods and problem-centred methods. The emotion-centred methods help you feel better even though you are being discriminated against. These methods do not lead to improved employment-related outcomes although they usually help individuals feel more empowered while enduring discrimination.

Problem-centred approaches involve either taking proactive steps that may help to reduce the level of discrimination or reliance on a specific job or, when all else fails, using legal means to address discrimination. Proactive steps involve the use of strategies that may be successful in partially alleviating discrimination. These strategies often facilitate success in most work situations, so they are good career-building steps in any case. They include creating a persona of success, securing additional training and taking good care of yourself via a lifestyle approach such as the OMS lifestyle. Experts often recommend securing additional education since it increases employability and makes people less dependent on what may be a poor employment situation. Additional training can offer opportunities to move out and up.

One factor often overlooked is image. Studies consistently find that attractive individuals rise higher work-wise and earn more than less-attractive individuals. This does not mean that individuals have to be as attractive as movie stars. Instead, 'attractive' means looking healthy and appropriately well groomed. Paying attention to image is wise especially when confronting discrimination.

There are strategies to deal with the discrimination that people with MS may face at work

If none of these approaches works, there are usually other opportunities or legal options. Many countries have laws related to discrimination and have agencies that can investigate and address complaints of discrimination. Lodging complaints with government agencies may also be an option. Complaints may cause employers to reflect on their hiring and workplace practices and change their ways. Pursuit of legal remedies needs to be carefully investigated and considered, as these are not always successful, so it is sensible to approach their use with forethought and consideration of costs involved. The courts in some jurisdictions are quite supportive of those seeking correction of discrimination while others rarely rule in favour. Before spending time, money and energy on discrimination lawsuits, it is important to understand the chances of succeeding. Sometimes local MS societies can provide some free advice on the best course of action.

For more discussion of disclosure and discrimination-related issues, see the next chapter, Chapter 15, by a lawyer with MS, Greg Hendron.

Sophisticated steps for overcoming discrimination

In addition to the basic techniques for overcoming discrimination discussed there are also techniques recommended by experts in leadership and organisational change. These steps have been developed in the fields of organisational communications and sociology.

A whole body of knowledge relating to leadership emergence discusses techniques that can not only help you to overcome discrimination but also make you a person to whom others turn for leadership. Research in this field has found that certain types of individuals emerge as leaders again and again. Those who emerge as leaders generally do two things: work harder than others; and care more about the group than others. Anyone can do these things. Anyone can make it a point to be supportive of others (as opposed to being critical) and to take time to help others when needed.

It is also prudent to pay attention to what sociologists know about social change (in this case, overcoming discrimination). Social change typically occurs when an innovator finds a champion—someone who occupies a higher-level position and will support and endorse the adoption of change. Accordingly, if you are having problems with discrimination, it is wise to seek a person in the organisation who can offer advice on what to do and also provide support. This development of a relationship with one or more champions is far more effective than engaging in self-pity or commiserating with others who are also victims of discrimination but who have little power to effect change.

When seeking champions, remember that most individuals like being asked for help and advice. One of the best ways to begin establishing a relationship with a potential champion is to ask for advice and to be appreciative when advice is given.

If you find that a champion is not available in a current organisation, champions from other organisations can assist. These people can help you to find new opportunities and avoid becoming stuck in a poor situation.

Networking

A good overall plan for addressing discrimination involves looking beyond a current employment setting by networking and expanding access to other opportunities.

Networking can be done in many ways. Many join professional organisations and use leadership skills to contribute to these organisations and earn the support and respect of others in the organisations. This can lead to employment opportunities.

Likewise, volunteer service in community organisations and use of leadership skills in community settings can lead to new opportunities. I have served on non-profit boards, volunteered as a political campaign treasurer, written campaign literature, overseen the bank accounts of a much older friend who was worried about being forgetful, sent a lawyer friend to visit the local jail to see someone who had been unjustly accused of a crime, solved neighbours' mobile (cell) phone and computer problems, done the shopping for a friend who didn't have transport, and many other things. I never know what someone in my networks will need but I always help when I can. In exchange, I often receive heartwarming help from others. Research shows that individuals like to help those who help them and they like to return favours. This is called reciprocity. When building a career, this knowledge can help you to cement good relationships with others and deftly avoid discrimination.

All effective networking efforts involve establishing authentic and sincere relationships with others; asking for advice, a contact or help if you need it; and generously providing the same to others when you are asked. Effective networking requires trusting others and generously sharing contacts even when you might not know someone all that well. Many employment positions are secured via contacts made through networks.

In summary, be proactive in addressing discrimination. Using the steps suggested here, such as advancing education and training, exercising leadership behaviour, and being a good friend and networker, can help insulate people from discrimination when it appears.

MS symptoms and work

Finally, let's turn to MS symptoms in the world of work. Researchers have identified two physical problems that predict work outcomes for people with MS: fatigue and extent of physical disability.

By far, the most common reason individuals with MS leave the workforce or reduce their working hours is fatigue. Many with MS simply feel too tired to work a regular job. With its emphasis on proper nutrition, exercise and psychological wellbeing, the OMS Program can help prevent fatigue. It can also help prevent other problematic MS symptoms, such as numbness and tingling, difficulties walking, general aches and pains, loss of motor skills, weakness and problems with heat. Many find that the Program by itself can eliminate most if not all symptoms within a few years, and others combine lifestyle improvements with MS disease-modifying therapies.

When it comes to physical problems as a result of MS the most important factor involves the amount of disability. In general, those with no visible disabilities are far more likely to be employed and well paid than those with visible and severe disability. At this time, best estimates are that about 80 per cent of those with no visible MS symptoms are employed while less than about 10 per cent of those who are not mobile are employed.

In general, the greater the degree of disability, the more problems occur in securing employment and comparable wages. However, even this factor is moderated by other factors such as education. For example, a physician is likely to be well paid and work until a regular retirement age even with visible walking issues. This means that even those with some significant disability issues can often find ways to secure satisfying and rewarding careers, given that MS typically affects young adults. Education opens doors to opportunities.

If you have visible MS physical problems, remember that there are often ways to mitigate their negative impacts on employment. Be persistent. Don't give up. Addressing physical problems aggressively using lifestyle improvement measures such as the OMS Program, physical therapy, and regular sleep often leads to the disappearance of many symptoms.

When first diagnosed, some may have a flare-up of symptoms that is severe enough that they must take time off work for a few weeks or months. Such temporary leave can often be negotiated with employers, and most individuals, especially if they make lifestyle improvements, are able to return to work within a few or several weeks. Within a few years, many find that they can go years and years without relapse.

A skilful healthcare team can help people with MS cope with the physical problems that arise from the disease. Your doctors can order physical therapy when needed, various tests to help better understand physical problems, tests to ensure your diet includes important nutrients, and so on. For help putting together a good healthcare team, see Chapter 11, Dr Heather King's 'Choosing your healthcare team'.

Importance of the OMS Program

Following the OMS Program is likely to be one of the best things you can do for your career. Eating a plant-based wholefood diet and exercising can improve mood, assist with weight loss if needed, provide more energy, address some MS-related emotions, help to prevent and alleviate employment discrimination, and help you to stay fit and ready to do an excellent job. It is a mistake to not follow the OMS Program and thereby to not be as healthy as possible.

Clearly the OMS Program will not solve MS-related problems overnight, or for everyone. It seems to take up to five years for some individuals to feel their best after they start following the Program. You may need to factor that time delay into your career-related decision-making. Many, of course, experience significant improvements much more quickly. In my own case, for example, all of my relapses stopped within one year after changing my diet and taking vitamin D3 on a regular basis. Research shows that those who cope most successfully with MS quickly make a decision to be proactive and show a stubborn determination to do whatever is necessary to improve the course that MS will take. Indeed, many who adopt lifestyle improvements live to very old age with minimal disability.

Healthy lifestyle is critical to maintenance of good health and, in turn, employment

In summary, following the OMS Program faithfully, taking advantage of educational opportunities, being persistent, and practising good leadership and networking behaviours are key.

Ground covered

Some important issues arise for people with MS who work. In the past, many with MS did not continue working until late in life because of disability issues. Thanks to improved approaches to treating MS that include lifestyle improvements, many now work until regular retirement age and beyond.

While a multidisciplinary approach is most effective in addressing some problems relating to work such as discrimination, it is sensible to adopt lifestyle choices such as the OMS Program as the basic foundation for other steps that can help improve long-term employability in meaningful and satisfying careers. The Program can help to prevent and alleviate physical symptoms associated with MS, address psychological issues that can arise with an MS diagnosis, make additional education possible and even help address employment discrimination. Other effective strategies for addressing employment-related issues include securing additional training, practising persistence, and improving interpersonal and networking skills to avoid being trapped in undesirable positions.

My Story: Anthony Mennillo

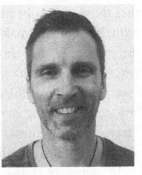

The year 2008 was a difficult one for me. I could feel my body getting sick. I couldn't focus out of my left eye and then pins and needles up and down my legs began and persisted. Numerous tests and MRI scans followed and on 24 July 2008, two days before my 34th birthday, I was told that I had MS.

It is hard to describe the sense of hopelessness and despair that I felt at the time. It took me about nine months to battle through the devastation of the diagnosis, the shame that I felt and the fear of what I thought my future would look like. I then stumbled upon the OMS Program. I read Professor Jelinek's book *Taking Control of Multiple Sclerosis* and in 2009 I attended an OMS retreat. At first this was very challenging for me because there were a few people attending who were quite disabled by MS, but by the end of the week I felt deeply inspired by their courage and determination to do whatever it took to improve their lifestyle or remain active.

The OMS Program and the inspiring stories of those who had adopted it gave me a sense of new-found hope and helped to ease my fears about the future I had originally anticipated—I embraced the Program wholeheartedly. Initially the changes to my diet and the introduction of meditation into my lifestyle were challenging, but within months I started feeling better and the OMS Program became my new normal. My health became my priority and I made decisions about my lifestyle accordingly. Today I am fitter and healthier than I have ever been. I do not have any MS symptoms and have not had a relapse since 2008. As a busy professional in a stressful job, it was clear that my work style needed to change. My MS diagnosis was something that I kept very private and despite my initial reluctance to discuss it with my employer I confided in a few key individuals who were entirely supportive. Together we decided to reduce my work hours to a nine-day fortnight, which allowed me to maintain a better work-life balance.

I have also learned to manage the stress of my work better through meditation. Quite often I stop whatever I am working on and sit mindfully, observing my breath for a few minutes, or I go for a short walk outside to centre myself.

I now look at my life differently and have an extraordinary sense of gratitude for so many aspects of it. With that in mind, I wanted to find a way to give back to Professor Jelinek and the OMS team for what the OMS Program has done, and continues to do for me. In November 2016, 23 of my family and friends joined me to run the New York Marathon and along the way we raised a significant amount of money for the OMS charity.

MS changed my life but not in the negative way that I had anticipated when I was diagnosed. It led me to the OMS Program and the Program has given me balance—balance in every aspect of my life. I firmly believe this balance will keep me on the path towards remaining healthy.

15

Disclosure

Gregory Hendron

> When you become involved with your OMS Circle, they become part of your extended family, your confidants, your friends, and the ones who truly know the journey that you're on.
>
> *Sean Kressinger, Launceston, UK, OMSer*

Disclosure is defined generally as 'the action of making new or secret information known'. There are many structured forms of disclosure in the business, legal, medical and political arenas. Indeed, as a lawyer with some twenty years' experience I am proficient in and comfortable with the application of the law on disclosure—that is, the process of revealing evidence held by one party to an action or prosecution to the other party. In some legal matters it is compulsory; in others it requires the support of the courts and in certain circumstances there is a right to non-disclosure. The rules are established, the parameters are clear and so the process is pre-determined.

There is, however, a distinct difference between the application of a set of rules on disclosure in a legal setting and determining the parameters for a personal disclosure of a diagnosis of MS.

The first rule is that there are no rules

The broad position is that there are no hard and fast rules when it comes to disclosing an MS diagnosis. Perhaps it would be easier for many of us if there were—as with anything new we often find the path easier to navigate when we are given step-by-step guidance on what actions to take, their timing, pitfalls to avoid and processes to apply.

However, the MS disclosure process, by and large, is a deeply individual one and can vary significantly from person to person. In the following sections we will explore the decision-making process surrounding disclosure, in particular:

- when to disclose an MS diagnosis, if at all
- the extent of that disclosure
- to whom to make such a disclosure.

We will consider both the personal and broader benefits of disclosure and how to manage other people's reactions. Hopefully, you will come away with an appreciation of the power of shared understanding and increased knowledge to break down the MS stigma.

Deciding when to disclose an MS diagnosis and to whom

For the most part, the time to disclose the diagnosis, the extent of that disclosure and to whom you disclose are entirely up to you. I say 'for the most part' because there are some formal disclosure processes that may need to be followed; these are covered further on. Your disclosure process will invariably be a gradual one, and potentially a lengthy one, with perhaps a staged disclosure to various groups of people, personal to you or within the wider public.

My disclosure journey is perhaps one of the more protracted you will encounter. Indeed, it is particularly poignant for me that I have been invited to write this chapter on disclosure. While I was wholly comfortable with disclosure of my MS diagnosis in a professional capacity, I was ironically wholly uncomfortable with disclosure in a personal capacity—sharing my diagnosis only with my immediate family for the first six years!

For a long time I was fixated on the notion of returning to my 'old self' and consequently saw no need to disclose the MS diagnosis to anyone outside of my immediate family; my plan was essentially to reset both physically and mentally to my pre-MS state. However, life is a journey forward, not backwards—it is about experiencing, learning and progressing. As such our 'old selves' are exactly that, an old or former version of who we presently are.

Determining when to disclose a diagnosis of MS, to whom to disclose it and the extent of that disclosure is very much a personal process

Yes, the current me has been diagnosed with MS but that is not my defining characteristic. In accepting the diagnosis, disclosing the diagnosis and adopting the OMS Program, I am now the best version of myself.

It is only in retrospect that I can see the immense burden that non-disclosure placed on me, and the immense burden that I placed on my family in asking them to keep my diagnosis a secret.

Non-disclosure does not mean no discussion

Even though we may elect not to disclose our diagnosis to our broader social circle, our colleagues, professional acquaintances and the wider public, this does not preclude people from enquiring as to what is going on. It is human nature to wonder, speculate and discuss. Often, we and our immediate family or loved ones are faced with difficult questions from people we do not wish to disclose our diagnosis to yet, or at all. The type and level of questions vary depending on the personal/extenuating factors addressed below.

For example:

- if you have a long leave of absence from work, colleagues will ask why
- if you are displaying physical changes, friends will ask what is happening
- if you are unsteady on your feet in a bar or restaurant, staff or the general public may assume you have been drinking excessively.

Being in a position to address these issues directly and honestly is much easier than trying to sidestep them.

Variables and extenuating factors

There are many variable and extenuating circumstances that affect our disclosure journey. The disclosure process is an inherently personal one, just as the nature of each individual diagnosis is. There are factors specific to your diagnosis that may necessitate a more expedient disclosure approach. If you have experienced symptoms for many years and receive a 'late' MS diagnosis, you may have multiple and latent symptoms that make disclosure unavoidable or non-disclosure tricky. You may require a level of physical assistance that necessitates a fully transparent approach.

Supplemental to this is the type of support network that is available or that you want to avail yourself of. Where you have a supportive spouse or a close-knit family or friendship circle, you may feel that disclosure to them and them alone is sufficient in the first instance.

Where you receive an MS diagnosis but do not have these types of relationships available to you or do not feel that they are a suitable first port of call, you may look for support in other ways, such as:

- seeking solace by talking with others with a similar diagnosis and so in a position to empathise—perhaps by joining an OMS support group or local circle
- disclosing to a person or persons in your broader social circle
- seeking professional or counsellor guidance.

As well as the practicalities of diagnosis, arising needs and support network, our particular personality is very important in the disclosure process. Some of us need to tell everyone right away—to unburden ourselves, navigate the journey and understand how to move forward. For others of us it is a deeply private matter that we need to process personally, without the involvement of others.

Disclosure to specific groups

If you decide to disclose your diagnosis, there are broadly seven groups of people to consider:

1. immediate family members and loved ones
2. wider friendship circle and extended family

There are many variable and extenuating circumstances that affect our disclosure journey such as the nature of our individual diagnosis, the support network available and our personality type

3. employer
4. colleagues
5. formal organisations, public bodies and insurance providers
6. the general public
7. others with an MS diagnosis.

Disclosure to each of these groups may require differing approaches and invariably will yield different responses.

Immediate family members and loved ones

Perhaps contrary to popular belief, disclosing an MS diagnosis to immediate family members and loved ones can be the single most difficult step on the disclosure journey. The reasons for this are that:

- immediate family members and loved ones are often the first group of people to whom we disclose. The timing of such disclosure is generally very close to or immediately following diagnosis. This is a deeply dark, often despairing and difficult time for many of us, where we are facing an uncertain future framed by an autoimmune disease renowned for being degenerative, aggressive and incurable
- immediate family members and loved ones are deeply invested in our emotional and physical wellbeing and happiness, as we are in theirs, leading to heightened emotions all round.

This said, it has become clear to me that disclosing the MS diagnosis to immediate family members and loved ones is perhaps the single most important and beneficial step in the disclosure process. Why is this? It is fundamentally important that you feel supported and that you are not alone in the early days of an MS diagnosis. As such it is critical that you are able to lean on someone and where you have a supportive spouse or close-knit family circle, this seems the most obvious choice. They know you for exactly who you are, and so you can be candid and unguarded in their presence. However, while you can control the disclosure process, you cannot control the reactions of those to whom you disclose.

As noted previously, immediate family members and loved ones are emotionally invested in your wellbeing and tend to display a range of reactions from sympathy to shock, sadness to supportiveness and even, at times, frustration and resentment. As it is for you, the journey is new and daunting to them; like you they are trying to navigate it as best they can; and they may grieve the loss of what was.

Disclosing the MS diagnosis to immediate family members and loved ones can be both the single most difficult step on your disclosure journey and the single most rewarding one

My own disclosure journey has taught me that it is critical to deal with the feelings and range of emotions on both sides as a collective unit, with an open and forgiving mind, as and when they come. You may find, as I did, that you will witness strength, resilience, unequivocal support and love in your close circle. Invariably this will serve as a great source of comfort and encouragement in those critical early days as well as in the long term.

Wider friendship and family circle

Once you have disclosed to your immediate family members or loved ones, the process of disclosing to the wider family circle and friends should be an easier one. This is of course if you decide to tell them at all.

There are several factors for consideration when it comes to your wider family circle and friends. Depending on the circumstances, the wider family circle may have some knowledge or awareness that you have been 'unwell' for a time; they may ask your immediate family members or loved ones what the diagnosis is. You may decide to permit your immediate family members or loved ones to disclose on your behalf (to save you from having to do so) in a structured fashion (that is, they call around the family and let them know) or in an ad hoc fashion (that is, as and when they are asked). Alternatively, you may want to have those disclosure conversations yourself, to control the narrative and extent of disclosure.

The perceived benefits of disclosing to the wider family circle include:

- a more expansive support network
- it can unburden both you and immediate family members and loved ones—there will be no necessity to avoid difficult conversations, circumnavigate the truth, and so on
- as MS is a disease that runs in families, family members will have an opportunity to modify lifestyle choices and implement preventive measures as they deem necessary.

Similar considerations apply to the wider friendship circle. Often friends will wonder why you might no longer be socialising with them, perhaps why you have stopped coming to football, why you have been off work, changed your diet, and so on. Disclosing to them can similarly lead to an extended support network, the renewed ability to socialise with their understanding of new parameters or constraints, and an unburdening.

While the process can be a cathartic and generally a positive one, it is worth reiterating that you cannot control people's reactions. If you are faced with a negative reaction, maybe this is an opportunity to review the friendship and time for you to reconsider where that person fits in your life.

Employer

Disclosure to your employer may be either mandatory or discretionary. The categorisation will depend on the nature of the job, details of the contract of employment or any relevant health and safety or employment legislation. If you have any concerns or are uncertain of your position it is best that you take advice from an appropriately qualified third party. You may wish to investigate what local protections are in place to safeguard your employment following disclosure of a health condition. Similarly, many countries have laws to ensure that individuals with disabilities are provided with similar opportunities as other people for workplace access.

Whether disclosure to your employer is mandatory or discretionary, there may be additional factors that shape the decision of whether or not to disclose, including whether suitable adjustments will need to be made to facilitate a return to work and whether you are still equipped to fulfill your role.

There can be a real fear of disclosing an MS diagnosis to an employer. Some people with MS believe that both management and their colleagues will have a diminished perception of their capabilities and as a result treat them differently in the workplace.

Disclosure to an employer may be viewed as a high-risk strategy but at the same time may be viewed as a positive one. By making the diagnosis known it affords employers the opportunity to make reasonable adjustments, if needed, to ensure that you can perform to the required level. Colleagues will be aware of the diagnosis and will often do everything in their power to help. As a result, your workplace may become a more positive working environment, influencing you to stay long term.

It may be worth giving thought to a disclosure conversation with your employer, devising a strategy that:

- determines the extent of disclosure and provides an explanation of how it will affect your ability to deliver the job role
- allows you to bring to the table positive suggestions for facilitating a smooth and effective return to work.

Colleagues

Many people with MS will have had some sort of leave of absence from work. It is commonly felt that a diagnosis of MS can be very difficult to obtain and is often only given after significant neurological effects have been experienced—these usually manifest through physical changes, noticeable to family, friends and colleagues.

If you have disclosed your MS diagnosis to your employer and are returning to work, it is worth considering disclosing to colleagues, particularly where noticeable employer-level adjustments have been made to facilitate your return. As with your wider circle of family and friends, your colleagues will invariably have wondered and possibly even asked about your absence and illness. Colleagues will generally be supportive and accommodating so that your immediate return to work and continued employment is as stress-free, manageable and fluid as possible.

Formal organisations, public bodies and insurance providers

This is where the 'There are no rules' rule may fall away. There are myriad bodies regulating areas such as driving, medical cover, and insurance requirements that you may need to liaise with post-diagnosis, to ensure that your actions remain within the law or that you are not invalidating existing contracts or agreements. These will be specific to where you live and to the personal cover that you have taken for items such as health insurance, travel insurance and life assurance.

By way of example, I am a resident of Northern Ireland. The Driver and Vehicle Agency stipulates that it is mandatory to notify it of a diagnosis of MS and with this come shorter licencing periods and rigorous driving checks. Where you fail to notify, you are driving illegally. Many insurance providers within Northern Ireland require full medical disclosure with policy renewals; failure to disclose invalidates cover.

It is important that you check where you stand and take independent advice where there is any uncertainty. Notably, disclosing the diagnosis, via government or Inland Revenue sites, may give rise to entitlement to financial support. This will be particularly important where absence from work or discontinuation of employment has financial implications.

General public

You may ask why you would disclose your diagnosis to the 'general public'. In this respect we are not considering an all-encompassing announcement to the world for the sake of it but more so a 'practical' approach to disclosure where a situation or circumstance may merit.

We will all encounter situations where the ability to explain them away with a diagnosis of MS is by far the easiest option. Again, the extent and nature of this will depend on the severity and extent of symptoms. These are the sorts of situations where you may feel compelled to disclose:

- needing to ask for a seat on public transport
- explaining dietary requirements in a restaurant
- assuring staff in a bar that your difficulty walking is not the result of excessive alcohol
- getting assistance with baggage in a hotel.

Others with an MS diagnosis

Having to confront an MS diagnosis can be a harrowing and dark experience for many of us. MS is a disease that is renowned for being incurable and degenerative, usually leading to disability. Finding a program like the OMS Program will bring you into a community of people living well with MS who will inspire hope in you for the future.

Disclosing to others on the OMS journey enables you to benefit from a unique sense of empathy, one that is hope-giving and insightful

The OMS Circles and the online OMS Forum are unique as those participating in them can empathise in a way that our loved ones and wider circles cannot. They are on a similar journey, have learned lessons, seen progress and so have a unique perspective to share. You should most definitely consider disclosing your diagnosis to this community. The benefits can be immense.

Disclosure and unburdening yourself

While the idea of disclosing a diagnosis of MS may be extremely daunting, the benefits that disclosure can bring about are significant and as such worth careful consideration. Letting go of the 'secret' can lift a weight off your shoulders that you may not have realised you were carrying. The process can be massively unburdening and cathartic.

Go at your own speed, allow yourself time to heal, understand your needs and identify how you want to proceed

It may allow you to tap into a wonderful support network, aid your recovery and learning, and facilitate an easier transition back into everyday life. Do not rush the process, however—take it at your own speed and embark on it incrementally, allowing yourself time to digest the diagnosis, understand how you want to proceed and who you want to tell.

Disclosure and deconstructing the stigma

There is a limited amount of research in the area of disclosure and impact; that said, what is out there suggests positive results. Disclosure and discussion help to break down the stigma surrounding MS as an illness broadly regarded as degenerative, with the diagnosed person facing gradual physical and mental decline.

Sharing your stories of the OMS Program, hope, recovery or degeneration prevention with other people with MS can help the community's understanding of the illness, encourage others with MS and have a profoundly positive personal effect.

Ground covered

The process of disclosing an MS diagnosis is a deeply individual one. The journey will vary for each of us and will depend on a host of personal circumstances and preferences.

The critical considerations in respect of disclosure are twofold: one is making disclosures where it is mandatory to do so; the other is determining, where disclosure is at your discretion, to whom you wish to disclose, the extent of that disclosure and its timing.

In considering an approach to disclosure, it is important to prepare yourself for the impact it will have on you, for varying types of reactions and for any future repercussions.

While it is believed that many people with MS are reluctant to disclose the diagnosis, it is imperative to take heart from the fact that disclosing the diagnosis can in actual fact unburden you and yield positive results and support in both your personal and professional circles.

Your decision to disclose the MS diagnosis can have a profoundly positive effect for other people diagnosed with MS, especially once you start to share your experiences of living with MS and following the OMS Program, and help to dispel MS myths.

My Story: Professor Anne Kavanagh

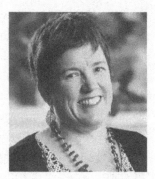

I was diagnosed with MS in August 2011 at the age of 48. I'd had unrelenting vertigo and problems balancing for six months. My daily 20-kilometre round-trip bicycle commute to work was taking fifteen minutes longer each way.

I am a medical practitioner and a professor in public health. I had rehearsed many different diagnoses, all of them involving something seriously wrong with my brain. I'd previously been admitted to hospital in 1990 with slurred speech and leg weakness but no definitive diagnosis was made, so I dismissed the symptoms as an 'inner ear problem' and lack of fitness. When I found the discharge letter from my 1990 hospital admission, MS was listed as a potential diagnosis but I'd forgotten about it. I am pleased I wasn't diagnosed with MS back then because I may have made different personal and professional life choices.

My 2011 MRI scan showed about twenty lesions consistent with MS. By the time I saw my neurologist my vertigo was constant and I wasn't able to walk far because my legs were so weak.

Disclosure wasn't really a choice for me because I had been so unwell at work and I returned to work using a walker after two months' sick leave. My colleagues were overwhelmingly supportive. I brought a camp mattress into work and slept in my office to manage my fatigue and clear my brain fog. I now work from home two days a week—actually full-time during COVID-19 lockdowns! Because I had an established career, I was able to negotiate the adjustments I needed to remain working.

Some family and friends imagined my life was in fast decline. My biggest challenge was dealing with the others' pity. I found myself reassuring people that I was still me—not a tragic version of my former self. Some good friends found it so hard they didn't contact me for months. I found myself trying to prove to others that I was the same as always, sometimes pushing myself beyond my capabilities.

A colleague who is a leader in the epidemiology of MS suggested that I attend George Jelinek's OMS retreat. Meeting George and fellow MS travellers brought me hope that there were things I could do to help myself. High-quality evidence on lifestyle interventions for MS is still accumulating. This contrasts with other chronic conditions like coronary artery disease where lifestyle interventions have been the cornerstone of management for decades. The OMS Program has offered me a way to bring what we know about lifestyle interventions for people with MS into my own life. I can't say I am perfect at it. I have a lot of stresses in my life and managing these in ways that support my wellbeing is a challenge.

My diagnosis has given me a greater appreciation of life. I love walking in the bush, swimming in the ocean, travelling to new places, taking photographs, and hanging out with family and friends. I also love my work. Nine years ago I wasn't sure I'd be able to keep doing these things. But I can.

16

Pregnancy and childbirth

Dr Keryn Taylor

> My husband, daughter and son-in-law follow the
> OMS Program with me; we are all healthier as
> a result . . .
>
> *Anne Atkinson, Derbyshire, UK, OMSer*

MS is a disease that is most commonly diagnosed in women aged
in their twenties or thirties, right at the time when many people
have started or are planning to start a family. A diagnosis of MS
can influence many decisions about starting a family, pregnancy,
delivery and parenting. For some people, MS can cast a shadow
over these decisions and experiences, bringing fears about their
future and the impact of MS on their ability to be a parent to their
children.

In fact, in the past many healthcare professionals actively discouraged women with MS from having a family. Fortunately,
the past 50 years have seen a dramatic shift in the understanding
of the period around childbirth (perinatal period) and how it is
affected by MS. Clinicians are now encouraged to actively discuss
family planning early as part of evidence-based care. The experience of people who embrace the OMS Program is also clear. There
is every reason for people with MS to be confident and hopeful
about the ability to be well, to have a family and to be a parent
who enjoys life now and can look forward to a future of good
health for themselves and their family.

This chapter is best read in conjunction with the web page on pregnancy and MS on the OMS website (https://overcomingms.org/about-multiple-sclerosis/ms-encyclopedia/pregnancy-and-ms), where there are many references to support the statements made here.

Starting a family

MS can influence the decision to start a family; it might bring a sense of urgency because of fears about future health and potential disability or it might cause a delay or even prompt a decision not to start a family. Alternatively, MS may be a positive driving force to start a family, motivating people to change priorities and reach for important life goals. Many factors will shape a person's decision to start a family and how they parent, and of course some of these factors will not have anything to do with MS. But if MS is influencing your decisions, it is important to access the best information, support and resources so that you can make a decision that is right for you, your partner and children.

Important information and support are available to help people with MS make decisions about their health and having a family

Will MS make it harder to become pregnant?

No. The good news is that MS has not been shown to reduce fertility, although about 15 per cent of the general population (with or without MS) have difficulty becoming pregnant and may consider in-vitro fertilisation (IVF). IVF causes hormonal changes that may affect MS, just as the hormonal changes of pregnancy affect MS. A medication used in some IVF treatments, gonadotropin-releasing hormone (GnRH) agonist, may increase relapse rates while taking the drug, but the evidence is less clear for GnRH antagonists. If IVF is not successful there is an associated risk of more relapses, as pregnancy reduces relapse rates.

It is important to note that the women undergoing IVF with these reported outcomes were not on the OMS Program. The medical

recommendation for everyone, with
or without MS, is to make healthy lifestyle changes to increase their chance
of becoming pregnant. Specifically,
both men and women are recommended to eat a healthy diet, exercise,
be a non-smoker, avoid alcohol and
reduce stress to improve the likelihood
of conception. These recommendations for everyone sound exactly like

*MS does not
reduce fertility
and the OMS
Program improves
the likelihood of
becoming pregnant
as part of a healthy
lifestyle*

those in the OMS Program. So, if you are following the Program
and are planning to start a family, you already have a head start
on giving yourself and your partner the best chance of success.

I am pregnant: will MS affect pregnancy and delivery of my baby?

Time for more good news. Generally, MS has little or no effect
on pregnancy and people with MS can expect normal pregnancy
outcomes, with no increased risk of adverse outcomes for mother
or baby. Women with MS do not have 'high-risk pregnancies' and
are at no greater risk of pre-term delivery, caesarean section or
forceps delivery. There are also no increased risks associated with
the use of epidural or spinal anaesthesia during delivery.

The OMS Program is likely to stabilise and improve MS activity
and reduce the likelihood of MS progression during pregnancy.
The Program can also reduce the risk of gestational diabetes, antenatal and postnatal anxiety and depression, pre-eclampsia and
pre-term delivery, and is likely to improve the overall experience
of pregnancy and delivery, all by virtue of promoting a healthier
lifestyle.

The delivery of a baby can be a time of excitement and
nervous anticipation. It is important to feel confident about
obstetric care and be informed about what is likely to happen
during delivery and postnatally. Your medical team may include
an obstetrician, midwife, general practitioner (primary care physician) and lactation consultant. A physiotherapist can help with

exercises to maintain and improve pelvic floor muscles during pregnancy and postnatally, particularly for people with MS who have symptoms affecting continence. Women may plan to have a vaginal delivery and this mode of delivery offers many benefits to mother and baby. There are also factors that can't be controlled, which may mean the delivery is not what parents had hoped for. Taking a mindful approach to pregnancy and delivery will serve people well in managing this time. Looking forward to the arrival of a healthy baby can be helpful in accepting and dealing with some of the challenges that can occur during pregnancy, delivery and the postnatal period.

Will following the OMS Program during pregnancy have any benefits for my baby?

Yes. Children may have a reduced risk of MS and overall improved neurological development. Another significant benefit is a lower chance of many other illnesses such as diabetes, rheumatoid arthritis, SLE, ulcerative colitis, asthma, dermatitis, breast cancer and mental ill-health. Research suggests that this lower risk may even be passed on to future generations.

MS does not increase the chances of problems during pregnancy and delivery; following the OMS Program provides significant benefits during pregnancy for both mother and baby

But will pregnancy affect my MS condition?

It is widely accepted that a woman's MS condition improves during pregnancy. The evidence is clear that during pregnancy there is an associated reduction in relapse rate, with a 70 per cent reduction in the third trimester. This is due to the well-established relationship between hormonal and biochemical changes of pregnancy and MS.

However, there is a possible increase in relapse rates in the first three months postnatally for some women who have high levels of disability and high relapse rates before pregnancy. This finding of increased relapse rates postnatally is not found in research on women with low levels of disability and low relapse rates pre-pregnancy. Despite this potential increase in relapse rate for some postnatally, the majority of women (around three-quarters) do not have relapses during this time. Stability of MS before conception is the best predictor of MS activity after the birth. Adopting the OMS Program before pregnancy and stabilising the disease is very likely to have a protective effect against MS activity postnatally, and the experience of women on the Program certainly supports this.

In the 3–12-month period postnatally, a decrease in relapse rates has been observed. The really great news is that there is evidence that in the longer term pregnancy may be beneficial for women with MS. Women with MS who have had children have lower long-term relapse rates, slower rates of progression to disability and a lower risk of developing secondary progressive MS compared with women with MS who have never given birth.

Pregnancy and childbirth have a positive and long-lasting protective effect against MS

Pregnancy and childbirth are also associated with a lower risk of developing MS and later age of onset of MS, giving more strength to the view that pregnancy has a positive and protective effect against MS.

Should I change my diet?

The OMS diet as outlined in this and other OMS books is excellent for women with MS during pregnancy and postnatally. It improves the health of both mother and developing baby during pregnancy and has immediate benefits for the newborn baby as well as lowering the risk of many illnesses for the child in the long term. Adopting a healthy diet is one of the best things you can do for yourself and your baby. A wholefood plant-based diet with omega-3, vitamin D and folic acid supplements is highly recommended.

Omega-3 supplementation during pregnancy can prolong high-risk pregnancies and improve birth outcomes for the baby, such as a healthy birth weight and enhanced visual acuity and neurocognitive skills. Omega-3s consumed during pregnancy reduce inflammation, improve immune function and are likely to reduce the risk of autoimmune and inflammatory diseases, such as asthma, allergy and dermatitis.

The OMS Program recommends eating fish and seafood, although this is optional. During pregnancy women who choose to eat seafood should limit the amount of fish they eat to avoid toxic levels of mercury. They should also avoid shark, marlin and swordfish and limit oily fish to twice a week. It is perfectly reasonable to avoid fish and seafood completely while pregnant and eat a plant-based diet with flaxseed oil. Following the OMS diet recommendations will provide all the healthy fats that are needed for the baby's development and wellbeing. Whereas a diet high in fat, particularly saturated and trans fats, is detrimental to both a mother and her baby's health, increasing the risk of anxiety in children, lowering the age of puberty and increasing the risk of breast cancer. These risks are all reduced when you follow the OMS recommendations.

The effects of what is consumed during pregnancy literally last a lifetime, if not longer. Mothers who eat a healthy diet while pregnant are likely to have children who naturally choose to eat a healthy diet and are also able to maintain a healthy weight. A mother's healthy lifestyle has clear benefits for her, her children and, through the process of epigenetics (the way our lifestyle influences the expression of our genes), even for her grandchildren. Embracing the OMS Program not only helps you to stay well but it can literally help to facilitate a much greater likelihood of good health for generations to come. What a gift to be able to give our children.

As pregnancy progresses, energy intake increases. Have healthy snacks such as fruit and nuts, and drink lots of water. Eating small amounts of food often helps to relieve morning sickness. There is no evidence that 'cravings' for specific foods while pregnant are caused by nutritional deficiencies; rather, they are a reflection of social influences. There are many excellent food ideas and recipes on the OMS website and in the OMS cookbook, which can provide great new options for foods to enjoy while pregnant. The body does require more iron during pregnancy; this can usually be met through diet or through supplementa-

A plant-based wholefood diet with omega-3 supplements during pregnancy is excellent for good health for mother and baby

tion. Vitamin B12 may be supplemented to ensure neurological development for the baby, particularly if the mother has chosen a plant-based diet with no seafood or fish.

Are vitamin D supplements safe during pregnancy?

Vitamin D supplementation is not only safe but essential during pregnancy for the health of both mother and baby. It is vital to supplement with vitamin D as recommended in this book and to enjoy time outside in sunlight when possible. Optimal maternal vitamin D levels are protective against MS activity in the mother, and reduce the risk of gestational diabetes, pregnancy-induced hypertension and low birth weight. A newborn baby's vitamin D level depends on the mother's vitamin D level during pregnancy. Babies born with vitamin D deficiency are not only at increased risk of MS but also a number of serious medical conditions, such as childhood asthma and respiratory infections.

Pregnancy is a key point in an unborn child's life where vitamin D supplementation can provide huge benefits. It's recommended that you check your vitamin D level prior to conception to ensure it is within the optimal range and monitor the level in the third trimester and one month

Vitamin D supplements are essential during pregnancy to protect against MS for mother and baby and for many other health reasons

postnatally. During the perinatal period there are a number of metabolic changes in the body that can reduce the level of vitamin D. If levels are low, consider taking a booster dose to quickly get the level above 150 nmol/L and increasing the daily vitamin D dose.

If breastfeeding, the mother's vitamin D level dictates how much vitamin D passes into the breastmilk. If the baby is not breastfed or once breastfeeding stops, supplement with vitamin D according to the OMS recommendations for children—these are discussed in Chapter 9, 'Families and prevention'.

What is the effect of stress during pregnancy?

Associate Professor Craig Hassed describes how important the mind–body connection is for health in Chapter 6 on meditation and mindfulness. Not surprisingly, managing stress and looking after the mind–body connection during pregnancy are vital for the health of mother and baby. High levels of stress during pregnancy are associated with miscarriage, pregnancy-induced hypertension, and pre-term labour. For baby there is an increased likelihood of a number of poor outcomes, including diabetes, asthma, cerebral palsy, attention deficit hyperactivity disorder (ADHD) and autistic traits in childhood.

How can stress be reduced in pregnancy?

Chapters 12 and 13 in this book on mental health and building resilience provide excellent strategies that can be used throughout the perinatal period. Adopting the OMS Program and prioritising sleep and exercise while pregnant are great ways to reduce stress and look after mental health. Actively making time for enjoyable activities, practising mindfulness and maintaining social connections all help to reduce stress, whether stress is related to pregnancy, MS or other parts of life. If symptoms of anxiety or depression occur during pregnancy, speaking to a healthcare professional and engaging in psychological therapy can be really worthwhile.

Research examining the effect of reducing stress during pregnancy found improvements in the mother's sleep, level of comfort and mental health, as well as less diabetes and hypertension. Stress-reduction interventions are also associated with better birth outcomes, including fewer pre-term deliveries, shorter labour and improved birth weights.

Actively reducing stress across the perinatal period has many benefits for both mother's and baby's mental and physical health

Should I take MS medication before and during pregnancy?

It is difficult to research the safety of medications during pregnancy because of ethical issues around exposing a foetus to unknown risks. However, there is a lot of clinical experience with outcomes after women have inadvertently become pregnant while on DMTs, and some MS medications have been used in pregnancies without adverse outcomes.

Glatiramer acetate (Copaxone) is licensed for use during pregnancy and has no adverse effects. Interferon is associated with only minor adverse effects. Most MS medications are only recommended during pregnancy if the disease is very active and the benefit of the drug outweighs the associated risks.

Fingolimod (Gilenya) and natalizumab (Tysabri) should be stopped several months prior to conception due to the risk of miscarriage and malformations. Fingolimod in particular is likely to result in poor outcomes in pregnancy and women should use contraception while taking this drug.

In some cases where MS is highly active and due to the high risk of rebound activity when natalizumab is stopped, natalizumab may be continued during pregnancy but should be stopped by 34 weeks of pregnancy; blood abnormalities may occur in babies exposed to this drug in late pregnancy.

Other MS drugs lack safety data and are not recommended. Ocrelizumab should be ceased twelve months prior to conception and teriflunomide should be ceased two years prior to conception unless an accelerated elimination process is initiated by your doctor. As new drugs are coming onto the market regularly, we suggested checking the pregnancy page on the OMS website if considering starting a family.

A short course of steroids is generally considered safe for treatment of a significant relapse during pregnancy or while breastfeeding.

Is there any risk for the baby if the father is taking MS medications?

During pregnancy, the risks outweigh the benefits of most MS medications and they mostly should be stopped

Teriflunomide (Aubagio) is an MS medication known to affect men's sperm and consequently conception. A man taking teriflunomide needs to stop this medication for two years prior to conception. Glatiramer acetate and interferon beta are not associated with adverse outcomes in the newborn baby when taken by the father.

Please always discuss medication with your doctor for the latest advice, and see Dr Jonathan White's Chapter 7 on medication for more detail.

Breastfeeding and MS

Breastfeeding has many benefits for both mother and baby. Mothers who breastfeed for at least four months are half as likely to experience a relapse postnatally compared with women who do not breastfeed. The baby's risk of developing MS later in life is also substantially reduced. Breastfeeding is an excellent way to ensure that the baby receives vitamin D via breast milk, as long as the mother has ensured her levels are high, further reducing the risk of the baby developing MS. Breastfeeding provides the optimal nutrition for babies and reduces the risk of many other illnesses such as asthma, diabetes and dermatitis. Breastfeeding can also help to soothe a baby and provide opportunity for bonding.

Breastfeeding is not always easy and help is available from midwives, lactation consultants and maternal child health nurses. There are also breastfeeding support groups, and many countries have laws in place supporting a mother's right to breastfeed in public and at places of work. Breastfeeding may be difficult or impossible, or a break in breastfeeding may be necessary. Restarting breastfeeding after a break or taking up breastfeeding at any point even if you weren't able to start immediately after the baby's birth nevertheless provide health benefits. Breast pumps can be used to initiate and maintain lactation and to express milk for later use. The most commonly prescribed MS medication during breastfeeding is glatiramer acetate, which is not associated with any adverse outcomes.

Breastfeeding reduces the risk of relapse for mother and provides protection against MS for baby; breastfeeding is not always easy, but there are lots of ways to get support

Some MS medications are not recommended during breastfeeding and, if breastfeeding is not possible, there are dairy-free, plant-based formula milks available. Whether a mother breastfeeds or not, there are many options to ensure that the baby receives good nutrition and bonds well with their mother.

Becoming a parent

Becoming a parent is a time of great joy, learning and adjustment. Parents can have many expectations about what family life will be like. Family and friends may have expectations as well; in fact, there is no other time in life where people will give so much well-intended but often unsolicited advice. There is also an endless number of parenting books and online resources, and a huge range of approaches to parenting. The only people who can decide what parenting approach is right are the parents themselves.

It is important for people with MS to take really good care of their health at all times but especially during the perinatal period, and this means prioritising the OMS Program, as outlined in this book. Becoming a parent is literally a life-changing experience where a parent becomes responsible for the wellbeing of another life. The natural response is to put the baby's needs first and at times this will be essential. But it is not sustainable in the long term and all parents must prioritise their own health, aiming to find the right balance between their baby's and their own needs. By following the OMS Program and prioritising physical and mental health, a parent can stay well and be present for their baby. Looking after one's health and connecting with partners require an investment of time and energy. It may mean accepting help to care for your baby, but it is time well spent and is essential for self-care.

As a new parent, look to simplify life wherever possible. Discover new simple OMS food and meals, stock up on easy meals in the pantry and freezer, exercise with baby and practise mindfulness with baby throughout the day (and night!). Be flexible and find new ways to stay well on the OMS Program that work for you and your family. All new parents experience fatigue, especially during the time when a baby is establishing a sleep pattern through the night. No parent, with or without MS, can stay well without good sleep. Parents need to rest and sleep when they can, and also continue to exercise to boost energy. They say it 'takes a village' to raise a child and this can mean accepting help from a partner, family, friends or formal childcare services. Although being a parent with MS can bring specific challenges, it is important to acknowledge that all parents need help and support. No one should feel they have to do it all and do it alone.

During pregnancy, expecting parents can set up a 'phone a friend' arrangement with someone they trust. It can be very helpful knowing that you have someone available to call for help if and when needed. Friends, family and social connection are important during the perinatal period. Parents often find that connecting with other new parents can be helpful during this time. These supports are often coordinated through local community health organisations or can be found online; they include the OMS community, which has informal parenting support groups on OMS social media platforms.

There are many formal supports and resources available from parenting services and medical and health professionals whose services can be easily accessed online and in person. Postnatal depression is common for women and men, and is more common for people with MS. The OMS Program helps to reduce the risk of anxiety or depression during the perinatal period, but if significant difficulties arise, it is important

Parenting is one of life's greatest challenges and rewards; prioritising the OMS Program and accepting help benefit both parents and baby

to ask for help early; the family doctor is a good place to start. There are many effective ways to recover from postnatal depression and specialist services for perinatal mental health are available internationally. Chapters 12 and 13 on mental health and building resilience provide many suggestions for achieving good mental health.

Ground covered

There are many reasons for people with MS to feel confident about becoming parents. MS does not affect fertility, and pregnancy may have a long-lasting protective effect against MS progression. The OMS Program offers many benefits to people planning to become parents and for women with MS during pregnancy and postnatally. The Program provides many benefits for the baby's development too, in utero, postnatally and for the child's long-term health outcomes, including a potentially lower risk of developing MS and many other diseases.

While becoming a parent can be one of life's greatest challenges, with or without MS, it is certainly one of the most rewarding experiences and there is lots of help available if difficulties arise. Whether a parent or planning to become one, people with MS who embrace the OMS Program can take great confidence and pride in the knowledge that their healthy lifestyle may benefit pregnancy, perinatal outcomes, their own health and the health of their children.

My Story: Lisa Downie

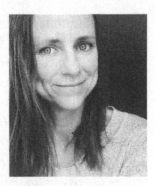

I was diagnosed with RRMS in October 2017. My first symptoms were slurred speech and dizziness that started suddenly one day at work. I had experienced strange bodily symptoms and a general feeling of unwellness on and off for a few years beforehand.

In 2017, a few weeks before I was diagnosed, I experienced an ectopic pregnancy, the result of natural conception after doing IVF for five years. After an emergency operation I was told that I was unlikely to ever have children; then, while still reeling from that, I was diagnosed with MS. A double blow so close together left me feeling empty, heartbroken and absolutely shattered. A few weeks after I got over the shock of the diagnosis, I started researching MS online and the OMS Program came up almost immediately. I had asked the neurologist upon diagnosis if I needed to make any dietary changes and I was told not to eat too much salt. That was it!

I started the OMS Program a few months after diagnosis. It took me a few months to get used to the idea of changing my diet and lifestyle. Once I did, I slowly said goodbye to my favourite non-OMS foods. Importantly, I no longer have the desire to eat these foods again. Finding the Program gave me back my sense of power, provided me with hope and put me back in the driver's seat, which are really important after such a big diagnosis and the feelings of helplessness and fear that immediately follow. It has also introduced new foods (hello nutritional yeast!) and new ways of cooking, which I actually really enjoy. I love the feeling of eating clean.

I attended an OMS retreat in November 2018 where I had the opportunity to meet others with MS. I realised how important it is to be able to connect with people who understand how you feel and who know what you might experience day to day. I left the retreat feeling empowered and it cemented the fact that the OMS Program was the right direction for me and propelled me forward towards a journey of healing.

And then in March 2019, you can imagine how thrilled I was to find out I was pregnant at 44, after having given up the idea of having children a year earlier. At the time I became pregnant I had been following the OMS Program for a year and felt healthier than I had in a long time. I felt amazing during pregnancy for the most part; there were a few times where I felt my old 'MS self', but it was only fleeting. Other than that, I had absolutely no issues during my pregnancy and also the postpartum period. Ziggy was born a very healthy baby.

I see the OMS Program as another form of medicine that helps to keep me well. It is the best possible thing that I can do for myself, my family and friends. I do find the diet the easiest part of the Program. It has taken a little longer to get used to meditation, or shall I say to keep practising it, even though it makes me feel so good. Having a baby has made it a bit harder to exercise and find the time for meditation, but I am slowly getting back into exercise and I make the time to meditate before bed. I still have bad days, but nothing sways me from the Program because I feel that it has given me so much.

As someone at my retreat said, 'Nothing tastes as good as healthy feels.' I couldn't agree more.

17

Sticking with the OMS Program

Dr Annette Carruthers

When your reason 'why' comes from within and is so powerful, you can achieve things you thought were impossible!

Anita Griffin, Cairns, Australia, OMSer

We all have a collection of major events in our lives when we remember where we were. My list includes the dismissal of Australia's Prime Minister Gough Whitlam in 1975, humans walking on the moon, and the deaths of John Lennon and Princess Diana. A more personal memory was in March 2001. I arose early and my right leg almost gave way on me. As a busy GP (primary care physician) I had patients booked to see me in an hour, so off to work I went. During the morning, my leg seemed to become weaker and I became increasingly concerned that it was a sign that something was badly wrong. After a quiet discussion with a GP colleague who agreed that there was real weakness in my leg and it was serious, I telephoned my favourite neurologist, also a family friend. It was 11 a.m. 'I'll see you at 2.30,' he said.

I was feeling very stressed at the time. It was a Tuesday. I was due to leave on an international study tour to the United Kingdom and United States on Friday and I was nowhere near ready. I had also been at a meeting the night before and enjoyed a Chinese meal with lots of deep-fried food and I had a tick bite on my arm. I also recalled an odd thing that had happened while bush walking the weekend before. I had fallen over on the trail. I had been mystified as to why that had happened.

The following day an MRI scan confirmed the diagnosis. It showed my first demyelinating (the myelin around my nerve fibres being damaged) event of MS. We know that many people with MS experience years of symptoms before the diagnosis is made. Sometimes there is even relief that the cause of ill health is identified. In my case, the worst days of my life followed as I quickly brushed up on MS and saw my dreams and aspirations evaporating in front of me. I calculated that based on averages, I would probably be unable to walk in sixteen years' time. I worried about my family and all the good times we had anticipated in the future.

I am forever grateful that my neurologist, after some thought, decided to postpone the introduction of disease-modifying medication until I had any further episodes. I now know that I could have spent years unnecessarily taking medications that carry a range of significant risks and side effects. Fortunately, my symptoms responded well to a short course of high-dose steroids (methylprednisolone) and physiotherapy. I returned to work after only two weeks, albeit at a slower pace. I am pleased to say that is the only time I have ever had off work for MS.

It was three weeks after diagnosis that a close friend told me they had heard about a recently published book, *Taking Control of Multiple Sclerosis* (first edn, 2000) by George Jelinek. George is medically trained and editor of a medical journal. It was a gift from heaven, offering as it did a comprehensively researched, logically argued, achievable approach. The Swank study published in the *Lancet* in 1990 on which George's dietary approach was based was so abundantly clear in its findings, I was convinced—and amazed that people with MS who could stick to a low-saturated fat diet remained largely well over 34 years! The sense of empowerment that George's book gave me—that I could now do something to try to keep myself well—was life-changing.

In the early days I didn't dare hope that I would remain well into the future by taking control, but as the months and years went by I had no further episodes. I am very grateful that I have been able to have a successful career, to nurture our two children and to travel extensively overseas. Nineteen years later I maintain the OMS lifestyle and live a full life.

The mind journey

The day of diagnosis was certainly one of the worst days of my life. It was so unexpected, such a shock. How does one come to terms with this? You can't continually live in fear of what might happen, what the future might bring.

The book *Anatomy of the Spirit* by Carolyn Myss was very helpful. It identifies how stress can cause and aggravate illness and how to recognise destructive thoughts, and make positive choices. My job as a doctor had already given me great insight into the role of stress in people's lives and the various ways that people respond to illness and approaching death. I knew that those who managed their health issues with calm, grace and wisdom had a better outcome and often a very spiritual and memorable experience of illness.

As a Type A personality, I had not really embraced the concept of meditation before. This meant that I had the most to gain by learning to relax and quieten my mind. The OMS retreats provided a great opportunity to begin to learn some skills. Another real benefit of the retreats was meeting people who had adopted the lifestyle some time ago and were doing really well, which was all very encouraging. I came away from my retreat feeling calm, empowered and with a stronger belief that the OMS Program was the way to go.

While I was reading *Taking Control of Multiple Sclerosis*, I was asked to take on a new patient in the local nursing home. She was a doctor, in her thirties and she had advanced MS. This was a very confronting experience. I gave her the very best care that I could, but it absolutely strengthened my resolve to do everything I could so as not to end up like this young woman, losing her career, her mobility and her independence.

Sticking to the OMS Program has been a journey. There have been many twists and turns over time. It hasn't been about sticking to a rigid lifestyle, but moving through a range of activities that came my way and that suited the time in my life. There remains so much to discover: new foods, new pursuits, so many valuable experiences to try. My wonderful friend next found a three-day Buddhist meditation retreat in a beautiful setting a short distance away, and we went together. In this setting we learned a range of meditation and yoga techniques, and yes, it became possible to gain a glimpse of the experience of nirvana, a place of perfect peace.

It is really important to be aware of your stress levels and to take time out for yourself to wind down. There is a wide range of hobbies and activities that can take you off the treadmill into a nice space. In the early days I undertook a photography course. Not only did I learn to take much better photos, but it really helped me see the beauty in the world, to appreciate an insect, a flower, an animal and a view. A walk now involves admiring native plants, noticing colour and light, and endless fascination with the nearby surf beach, lake and waterways.

Other pastimes that I have always enjoyed are sewing and knitting. As a young person I had made my own clothes. I do find the process of knitting or cross-stitching to be very meditative and I love creating new garments and undertaking really complex cross-stitch patterns. My current project of a Chinese vase and floral arrangement is the mother of all sewing projects that I have undertaken. Picking up the cross-stitch encourages me to relax but also focus the brain.

MS is known to affect cognition and this is a great concern. It's a powerful incentive to stick to the OMS Program. There is a theory of neuroplasticity of the brain—more simply put, 'use it or lose it'. It is important to keep the brain stimulated, by practising concentration and reinforcing memory, among other things. My work as a doctor requires continuing reading and education so I have no shortage of interesting information. There are many fun ways to stimulate the brain, such as learning a language, following concentration programs such as Lumosity and playing number games such as sudoku. All of these require a bit of a routine to ensure daily practice.

Embarking on formal study is another way to stimulate and test the brain. There are so many courses available for any interest. One fortunate outcome of the COVID-19 pandemic has been the conversion of many learning activities to the online environment. Through online learning another world opened up for me in the appreciation of classical music, by studying music history. I have gained immeasurable pleasure from this endeavour, not only in enjoying the vast array of wonderful classical music, much of it so beautiful and peaceful, but also in learning about the lives of composers over the centuries. I look forward to many more years of increasing enjoyment of music, closing my eyes and listening to Smetana's 'Moldau' or Mendelssohn's 'Fingal's Cave', such beautiful experiences. A very special piece is Elgar's *Cello Concerto in E Minor* played by Jacqueline du Pré. It is very powerful and uplifting and provides, given Jacqueline's own MS journey, inspiration to stick to the OMS Program.

Travel had always been an important part of our lives and there were many more places we wanted to see. This was a serious reason to stay well. Initially a family beach holiday was an achievement and after several of these went well we set more ambitious goals. Early overseas travel required much planning. This started with reading travel insurance contracts carefully and seeking cover that recognised pre-existing illness and having a management plan, including travelling with prednisone to take in high doses if another episode happened away from quality medical care. The sense of triumph I felt as the plane took off and we were on our way was a real reward for all the changes I had chosen to make.

The ability to travel was an incredibly important driver for me, and each successful trip reinforced the value that I was obtaining from the OMS Program

It was also really important to stick to the OMS diet while travelling as we certainly didn't want anything to go wrong overseas. Many holidays offer the advantage of increased exercise and plenty of sunshine. Sailing in the Mediterranean ticked all the boxes, with a wonderful seafood and fresh fruit and vegetable diet. Asian countries in general are also easier in terms of diet, with plenty of seafood and fresh vegetable dishes and marvellous tropical fruit. My favourite for the OMS diet was Japan, with its exquisitely presented seafood, sashimi and sushi; just hold the fried food. The worst country for the OMS diet was the United States. The prodigious food chains often serve incredibly fatty food with the ever-present accompaniment of fried chips. Even the salads are often doused in creamy sauces. Sometimes it took quite some searching to find a restaurant with appropriate food. I came to feel that if you lived there, you'd have to frequent farmers' markets and cook a lot at home.

If all else fails, when you are travelling, don't give in and eat fatty foods. There's no harm in grabbing some fruit or missing a meal and it's better for maintaining one's weight, too. In some countries the offerings can be quite limited and the food becomes repetitive, and if you are travelling in a group it is depressing to watch the rest of the party indulge while you are being careful and eating the same few dishes over and over again. Despite the negatives, I forever value the experience of having visited those countries. As time went on, we became more ambitious and I am pleased to say that our exploits have included Antarctica, Bhutan, Galapagos and Machu Picchu in Peru. Every trip I thank my lucky stars that I'm okay.

The exercise journey

Very early in my MS journey I began tai chi. A patient of mine was an instructor and over the years he had extolled the virtues of tai chi to me. He was delighted when I enrolled in his class. Tai chi is a series of slow and gentle exercises that require balance, coordination, concentration and commitment. It was perfect. The traditional Chinese movements are beautiful and accompanied by relaxing Chinese music. The concept of moving energy around your body (qigong) was empowering for limbs that had lost some strength. Each week I added some more movements, focusing the mind and building to a full routine. I was able to improve my strength, flexibility and balance and have a lovely relaxing meditative experience. I greatly appreciate the skill and dedication of my septuagenarian patient, who had dedicated so much of his life to introducing tai chi with all its benefits to so many people. Tai chi can be a program for life. Age is not a barrier and routines can be tailored to any disability.

I am fortunate to live near a beautiful deserted beach just twenty minutes from the city. Before my diagnosis, I would regularly walk to the beach, then the full length of the beach and back with my neighbour: a total of 11,500 steps once or twice a week. Each walk was a special experience, a communion with nature. No two days were ever the same at the beach due to the wind, waves and tide. I would often take pictures when it looked particularly spectacular, and I had done just that the weekend before I became unwell. I worried and wondered whether I would ever be able to walk that beach again.

In my exercise journey, I believed that effort would be rewarded and that improvements would keep coming for months and even years

I got my best photo of the beach framed and it became my inspiration to become strong again. From the first tentative steps with the physiotherapist, I knew I would have to work hard with rehabilitation to regain as much mobility as possible.

In addition to doing tai chi, I started doing some home-based exercises that helped and then it was time for the gym. I joined a local gym initially, using machines within my limits. The treadmills and cross trainers were really good for improving co-ordination, allowing me to walk more normally. Over the weeks I was gradually able to increase the weights and repetitions. It helped to record my progress as the weight that I was lifting increased, and eventually I was confident enough to begin pump classes. Pump classes help to build strength and coordination. The discipline of a class pushes you along, more than self-directed exercise does. The gym was a good experience: I met some new people there and a soak in the pool afterwards was a great reward.

The benefits of combining tai chi with the gym were that I could gradually walk further and further and that gave me the impetus to keep pushing myself. Walking to the beach became possible again and to this day every time I put my feet on the sand, I appreciate just being able to go there. Nature walks have become a favourite, with frequent trips to local national parks and even the Bay of Fires in Tasmania.

Water has always been an important part of my life and I knew that swimming was a great exercise for all ages. The local council began heating the pool and opening it year-round. At first I took some tentative laps, gradually increasing over time, adding different strokes for variety until I was comfortable swimming 2 kilometres. As at many pools, a social adult squad met three mornings per week with a trainer. They were a delightful non-judgemental group of all ages, with some amazing octogenarians. The camaraderie was an added benefit. The slow lane was perfect for me and being pushed by a trainer meant I received greater benefits from the exercise. While the tai chi and the gym have been replaced by competing priorities, swimming has become an essential part of my life. Two to three times per week, all year round, I have my swims, my sunlight exposure and even some meditation as I count the laps down.

The food journey

Anyone embarking on the OMS Program must experience those first realisations that some of one's favourite foods will be no more. My worst grief reaction was for cheese. However, it was very apparent that the OMS diet is a very healthy diet, not only for MS but for heart disease, cancer and mental health. There were a lot of benefits to be gained.

I was a foodie, I loved wining and dining. I loved to cook for dinner parties and entertain at home. The great news was the wine could stay! I have to say, though, I wasn't particularly fond of fish and, while my husband loved nothing more than a big serving of fish and chips, I worked on finding suitable sauces to disguise the taste of the fish. It is quite extraordinary how one's sense of taste can change over time and now I love nothing better than a piece of salmon or barramundi cooked to perfection. I knew that it was important for my children to increase their intake of seafood so I tried to make many meals that we could all eat, but these were interspersed with meals of their usual foods.

Local farmers' markets are a great source of a wide range of fresh and organic produce. I try to make a weekly pilgrimage, interacting with producers and artisans, purchasing what's in season and suitable for the OMS diet. These days I appreciate and enjoy the flavours of many more OMS-recommended foods than I did in the past. It's possibly also because fresh market produce is superior to foods kept for weeks and months in cold storage. Every time I discover something to assist with my cooking and enjoyment of food it's a new triumph. One of the best early finds was macadamia butter, which simply consists of ground macadamia nuts. Over the years it has become more readily available at farmers' markets and now I even have a local supplier.

It was only more recently that I discovered that homemade soy yoghurt is a good substitute for ricotta, crème fraiche, Greek yoghurt and buttermilk. This opened up an extraordinary range of possibilities, particularly in cake baking. I enjoy serving winter fruit puddings as a dinner party dessert from a recipe that includes macadamia oil, egg whites, ground almonds and soy yoghurt.

Fish markets are an absolute wonderland, offering an extraordinary range of fresh seafood. They are one of my favourite places to visit. There are myriad OMS-friendly recipes that can be made by substituting chicken with tuna, salmon or white fish. The OMS cookbook has also provided me with a range of creative food ideas that will take years to explore. Thank you so much to the people who compiled such a wonderful resource.

On reflecting with my close family and friends, a very important step for them was reading *Overcoming Multiple Sclerosis*; it really helped them understand what was required and how important it was for me. That meant I could happily visit their homes for meals and know that they would serve foods I could eat and enjoy. Spending time with my family, especially my siblings and their families, has always been a priority. They never questioned the changes that I have made and have accommodated them seamlessly, for which I have always been grateful. There have been many special Christmas gatherings where seafood, colourful salads

One useful tip is to invite family and friends to read Overcoming Multiple Sclerosis; *their understanding can make your journey much easier*

and my special Christmas cake recipe are traditional fare.

Eating at functions can be a greater challenge. For an office lunch I request a salmon salad sandwich (with no butter or cheese), or seafood sushi. Where individual meals are being served, it is always best that you inform the host of your dietary requirements. Initially I would advise that I can eat vegan and seafood, but after some embarrassing occasions when trouble was taken to make me a dish rich in coconut milk, I now include no coconut products as well. If I am staying anywhere for more than one meal, I provide a written note describing what I choose to eat, and what I choose not to. That approach makes it less daunting for those who are cooking for me. OMS now even provides a card that summarises the diet to hand out to restaurants.

I've been very thankful to the wonderful chefs who have prepared some amazing meals within the guidelines of the OMS diet. I am less than thankful to the lazy types who provide me with a dessert of the three melons (watermelon, honeydew and rockmelon) while my colleagues enjoy some delicious creation. This is balanced by the many occasions when my friends look on enviously as I devour a delicious dessert that was not on the menu and puts their sugary offering to shame!

There are always curious people who want to know why you are on the diet. I make it clear that it is very important for my health, without providing specific information.

Of course, I am often tempted to just eat things I used to really like. Yes, I have tried Portuguese tarts in Portugal but had more fun searching for the perfect sardine, prepared in a wide variety of ways. One strategy when tempted is to try an extremely thin slice of a special birthday cake or a favourite cheese, enough to appreciate the flavour but not enough to cause harm. At the end of the day, the person that you have to answer to is yourself. 'Cheating' yourself only puts your own wellbeing at risk and that's the bottom line. It's up to you to look after yourself and indiscretions should be very infrequent.

My husband and I loved dining out, and it was an important part of our lives before I was diagnosed. We've had lots of food adventures as we have travelled extensively. Locally it is always good to go to a seafood restaurant, but absolutely avoiding the battered and fried food. Most Asian restaurants also work well. Over the years it has been wonderful to see trends in restaurants move to more healthy eating, with offerings of lovely fresh salads and stir fries. One of the traps to be aware of are vegan restaurants, as many meat and dairy substitutes can be very high in saturated fat.

Even brunch can be a triumph, with egg whites, avocados and homemade baked beans (no meat, though). Eating out, I try to view the menu in advance just to be sure that there is something suitable for me. It is incredibly demoralising to find yourself somewhere where there is nothing appropriate on the menu. Most kitchens, however, are happy to make variations to meet your needs, such as serving the sauce on the side or holding the cheese, and those that aren't are certainly black-listed. If the dessert options are high in fat and there are no sorbets, there's always a delicious dessert wine!

The barriers

Having a close friend being diagnosed with MS and sharing her experience have reminded me of all the barriers and pitfalls along the way. In her case the neurologist simply stated that he didn't believe in the OMS Program, but that she could try the diet if she wanted to. He then handed her a list of a range of diets that she could consider trying. Over the years I've had a lot of contact with neurologists professionally and have been terribly disappointed by the attitude of many. They will tell you that there isn't enough evidence to routinely advise undertaking the OMS Program. From my point of view the Swank study was so definitive that it couldn't be ignored. There is now a very considerable subsequent evidence base that has accumulated, described in Professor Jelinek's books on MS or discoverable in PubMed, that our colleagues don't take the time to consider. Just type 'Jelinek G and multiple sclerosis' into PubMed (https://pubmed.ncbi.nlm.nih.gov/) and watch all the abstracts appear, and these are only the publications on the subject from one particular research group.

The reality of a lot of medical research is that there is much more funding for drug research than lifestyle changes. While lifestyle changes for heart disease and diabetes are very well established and encouraged, it is very disappointing that the same cannot yet be said for MS. These days there are an increasing number of neurologists who do recommend the OMS Program as part of a management strategy for people with MS. Probably the most encouraging point is that there is a significant cohort of medically trained people diagnosed with MS who have adopted the Program and have done extremely well on it. They know the consequences of poorly controlled MS and that's all the inspiration they need to make the appropriate changes to their lifestyle. A number of them are authors in this book.

It can be very challenging for people to stick to the Program when their doctors don't support it. It is also important to have family and friends support you. It was enlightening when a friend of mine was diagnosed with MS. Her family and close friends knew my story and almost insisted that she adopt the OMS diet. Her neurologist did not provide the same encouragement. When she told friends that she was undertaking the lifestyle changes of the OMS Program even though her doctor didn't believe in it, she received lots of disparaging remarks and very inappropriate suggestions on what to do. After a while she reverted to saying that her doctor had advised her to make the dietary changes and she subsequently received lots of support and encouragement to make the changes.

When I trained in medicine, it was believed that stomach ulcers were caused by stress and spicy foods. A very brave Australian physician, Dr Barry Marshall, showed that the bacterium *Helicobacter pylori* plays a major role in causing peptic ulcers and provided a breakthrough in curing this condition by medication. His theory was initially ridiculed by scientists and doctors and Dr Marshall has been quoted as saying 'everyone was against me, but I knew I was right'. Of course, he is now a winner of the Nobel Prize for his groundbreaking discovery. Another Australian, Dr Ian Frazer, developed a vaccine for human papilloma virus, now known to be a cause of cervical cancer. The vaccine is now predicted to eliminate cervical cancer in Australia by 2035.

Medicine is continually evolving and new conditions and disease management strategies are being developed for conditions such as HIV and now COVID-19. There are still no effective treatment strategies for the increasingly common chronic fatigue syndrome.

Just as an individual is on the journey of MS, so the medical management of this potentially debilitating condition also represents a journey

We need brilliant researchers who think laterally to help us to avoid the potholes and travel as well as possible through life. It is extremely frustrating that many of the major MS support and research organisations also fail to encourage lifestyle changes beyond general health recommendations such as stopping smoking and eating a low-fat diet with plenty of fruit and vegetables (but also allowing meat and dairy). The limited research on plant-based and seafood diets by the MS organisations is generally encouraging. The sad fact is that one day major medical authorities will accept the benefits already identified in non-drug research, and the advice will change, too late for too many people with MS. But of course, none of us has to wait. We can begin the OMS Program any time, for ourselves, without any outside oversight or indeed interference.

Upon asking a close friend to reflect on my journey, I received this response: 'You have been fully committed to the [OMS] diet over a long period. I think this relates to your belief in the rationale of the diet, and your faith in the doctor who developed it, but also to your continued lack of disease progression, which is positive feedback for your effort. You seem to enjoy finding alternatives that please your palate for those food groups you aren't recommended. I'm sure your professional understanding of how dire the outcomes of MS can be helps with your commitment as well.'

My brother has identified in my journey these features: 'A strong emphasis towards pursuing diligent research and clear decision-making, an appreciation of relevant recreational activities (e.g. swimming, walking and sailing), and maintaining a healthy relationship with food and drink and respective social opportunities based on food and wine appreciation. Also, much family engagement and encouragement of social gatherings and relaxing close to nature and appreciating the natural habitat.' Wise words indeed and not a bad prescription for a happy and healthy life for anyone, MS or no MS.

Ground covered

It remains up to each of us to make our own assessment of the available evidence underpinning the OMS Program and then embark on what is a lifelong journey to give ourselves the best chance of remaining well. It is not a great burden to protect and maximise wellbeing for the only life we have. While authority figures can sometimes undermine our efforts at such self-care, the OMS Program remains one that we can initiate ourselves and stick to ourselves, without outside help or interference.

My Story: Johanna Lahr

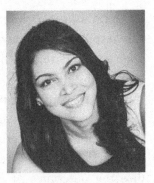

I have been living with MS since 2008; I was diagnosed when I was just at the peak of my professional and personal life. In 2002 I had started working in my dream company in a biotech department and I honestly loved my job. Up until then, I had lived a 'normal' life having had a happy childhood and no indications of what my future would hold in regards to my health. I am married and have a daughter.

In 2006 I was diagnosed with viral meningitis. Fortunately, I came through the worst and got better. However, I soon started developing a series of autoimmune disorders, MS being one of them. In 2008 I was prescribed my first course of steroids. In 2010 I had a bout of optic neuritis and I developed many other difficult symptoms. That year was no walk in the park. I was plagued with very painful sensory symptoms, 'MS hug', and fatigue, which I found very debilitating. I had difficulties coordinating simple functions like swallowing and breathing. My eyes were bad after several relapses over the year.

One day during a visit to a local neurological research centre I heard for the first time the name Jelinek. One doctor working there whom I knew from work told me to check out the work of Jelinek in Australia. I of course did! There was so much condensed wisdom in what I was reading. No frills, pure science. I ordered the *Overcoming Multiple Sclerosis* book and started immediately with all program steps and a plant-based diet. The OMS Program, enhanced by fasting and measures to protect gut health, became the cornerstone of my success. Just a couple of years after starting the Program I found myself relapse-free, mentally stable and financially independent. I realised that I had reached the long-dreamed MS remission.

But I had to face many obstacles and apply all of the lifestyle changes alone. It is true that to have the support of our loved ones is priceless but they can never understand what it is like to live with a chronic disease. I decided that I wanted to help other people with MS to learn about the OMS Program and give back a little of what I received. The Program literally gave me my life back. So I joined and started administering the OMS Lifestyle Support group on Facebook. Today, there are over 4500 members in this group. I have been leading the OMS Circle in Berlin, Germany, since 2018.

The importance of being part of a community should not be underestimated. It is not only a way to cope with the struggle caused by chronic disease; as OMSers, you feel like you don't need to re-invent the wheel on a daily basis. New habits, new techniques and strategies can be passed along from one OMSer to the next. Online community groups like mine that allow you to connect with people from all over the world are an endless source of wisdom, support and friendship from people who truly get it. Community can be so powerful.

Part 4

The road ahead

18

Facing an uncertain future

Karen Law

> The OMS Program offers me a blueprint to be a healthy human who just happens to have a diagnosis of MS.
>
> *Rachel Knight, Hawke's Bay, New Zealand, OMSer*

Life, by its very nature, is unpredictable. No matter how carefully we plan, there is always the chance that something unexpected will come along to change things. We learn that from a young age. Perhaps we've invited our friends to our child's birthday party at the local park but on the day there is a storm and we have to cancel. Or we're driving off on holiday with our family and all of a sudden a stone flies up and shatters the windscreen and we have to stop somewhere overnight and get it fixed. Natural disasters, accidents and random luck all have a role to play in our lives. We understand this and we accept it. There's nothing to be done.

When it comes to our bodies, however, the vast majority of us can rely on our arms, legs and brains to function predictably. We learn that from a young age too. As soon as we take our first tottering steps we find that we are able to do it again the next day and the next. Physical movement is a given and we come to trust in it completely. We know that when we stand at the edge of the road ready to cross we will be able to get to the other side before the cars come. We don't question it by asking, 'I wonder if my legs will make it this time?' because we're sure that they will. When we set off to climb mountains, hike trails or ride bikes we trust that we will have the physical and mental capacity to complete the tasks without exposing ourselves to undue risk. Function is automatic, predictable and taken completely for granted. We also understand that problems with our bodies, if and when they occur, are short-term. Broken bones mend, bruises disappear, wounds heal.

A diagnosis of MS appears to change all that.

Coming to terms with an unpredictable future

MS is rather unique in that the typical experience of people with the illness differs widely from one person to the next. Unlike heart disease, diabetes or Parkinson's, which operate in similar ways on the bodies of those who have the illness, MS comes with a wide range of symptoms and no two people's journey with the illness will look the same.

As we have seen in earlier chapters, damage to myelin can happen anywhere within the central nervous system; the resulting effect can therefore be felt in any one of a range of places in the body, affecting muscle tone, coordination, speech, vision, balance, bladder and bowel control, memory, mood, reasoning, sensation and pain. When you add to this the fact that relapses can occur at any time, without warning, it is easy to see why MS is believed to be one of the most life-altering diagnoses one can receive.

No wonder then that much of the literature provided to people diagnosed with MS refers to the need to adapt and make adjust-ments to take into account this new reality. Plan for the unexpected, we are told, accept your limitations, be prepared to transition to a new way of living. Taking control, in this literature, usually means approaching your situation with positivity and humour, finding a way to cope with the difficult position that you find yourself in.

It is this random, unpredictable nature of MS that causes much of the anxiety and fear associated with the illness. After 20, 30 or 40 years of completely reliable service our bodies, we are told, are now liable to let us down at any moment. Embarrassingly, dangerously, painfully. We can feel as though a time bomb is always ticking as we are left waiting for the next unexpected explosion of symptoms.

But does it have to be like that? For a short time, perhaps, but in the long run, no, for the majority of people it doesn't.

Early adopters of the OMS Program led the way

When sailors first set out to circumnavigate the globe, they had to put their faith in science as they had no personal experience to reassure them that the earth was in fact round. As more sailors made such trips and returned home safely, so it became easier for others to trust the science too and follow in their wake.

The first adopters of lifestyle management for MS were like these early sailors, trusting the science, as they had little or no personal experience to guide them. One thing in their favour, however, was the risk-free nature of the treatment. If diet and lifestyle modification turned out not to help MS, at least it couldn't possibly do any harm. Compared to the frightening prospect of sailing off the edge of the world, this was a pretty easy risk to take.

The first adopters of the OMS Program were pioneers; one big advantage of what they advocated was that it was and remains risk-free

As we have seen from the stories of several contributors to this book, the results of following the OMS Program turned out to be overwhelmingly positive for the first adopters. As more and more people began to experience the positive effects of lifestyle modification, a new literature started to emerge. This in turn encouraged a greater number of people from all over the world to adopt the OMS lifestyle.

Still, for any individual receiving a diagnosis of MS, and in the face of what is still a predominantly negative and disempowering picture of the illness, it can take a lot of faith to stay on course through the initial weeks, months and years. Our friends and relatives, albeit well-meaning, can often put us off from even trying to affect our outcome with MS such is the dominant paradigm that sees it as an incurable degenerative illness.

An optimistic view is a realistic one

Contrary to much of the MS medical literature, it is perfectly reasonable to adopt a generally optimistic outlook after a diagnosis of MS. In fact, it will almost certainly improve your outcome if you do. A pessimistic view will likely lessen your resolve to make the necessary changes, lowering your mood and overall quality of life. If you believe that your attempts will end in failure, why would you put yourself through the challenging process of changing your bad habits for good ones? So, optimism is important, but realism is helpful too. Knowing that it can and often does take between three and five years to stabilise the illness after making changes, we can expect some ongoing interference from MS even after adopting the most rigorous lifestyle changes. This can be hard to accept.

During the early months and years of the OMS Program it is helpful to see relapses and disease activity as part of the process to some extent. Since MS has often been active in the body for some time prior to diagnosis, and lifestyle change takes a number of years to reach full effect, it seems reasonable that a person will have to wait a while before experiencing the full benefit. It is helpful to have faith that the changes you have made are actually doing some good, even if you don't have concrete proof yet.

One of the major signs that the Program is working, especially for those of us diagnosed with relapsing remitting MS (RRMS), is a reduction in relapses. In the early stages it can be quite common to live with a feeling that another relapse is just around the corner. After all, that has probably been our lived experience of the illness so far. In time, however, longer gaps can occur between relapses until for many people they taper off altogether, often lessening in severity along the way.

Potholes on the open road

And so to a period of relative calm, after what is often a rather traumatic journey. The map can be put away, cruise control turned on, progress is constant, anxiety has abated, the future looks promising.

It's hard to overstate the sheer relief and outright joy felt on reaching this stage of the journey. Coming, as it often does, after a very difficult beginning with sometimes debilitating symptoms to contend with, accompanied by high levels of fear and anxiety. To emerge from this state and find yourself in a calm, confident place, with a body that is functioning correctly, or at least markedly better than it was before or no longer deteriorating, is truly a wonderful feeling. For many people MS becomes something that was in their past, a reference point for the way they live but with no actual meaning in their current life. For a great number of people this period lasts forever.

Achieving stability after a diagnosis of MS can be rightly viewed as a joyous outcome

Some of us, though, while cruising along this highway, will hit a pothole in the form of an unexpected relapse or sudden return of old symptoms. Sometimes this can happen after many years of complete stability. The fact that we are no longer expecting it can make such a pothole very hard to navigate. We are now cruising at speed, so hitting an obstacle is likely to have a much greater impact than if we were carefully nudging our way along a winding road as we were at the start of the journey.

Keep any setbacks in perspective

Many people panic when they experience an unexpected setback. This is understandable for two reasons. Firstly, MS symptoms are often unpleasant and disconcerting and it's hard to be sure where the relapse is headed or how serious it could become. Secondly, people with MS already have a pre-existing response to MS symptoms from their early experience with the illness. The discovery of a new symptom after a period of stable good health can throw us back to the same emotional place we were in on diagnosis: scared and anxious.

Probably the most helpful thing to do here is to keep things in perspective. If we adopted the OMS Program and managed to stabilise the illness after three years, then enjoyed four whole years of good health before experiencing another relapse or new symptom, this would actually still be a very good outcome. It is only when our minds start imagining that the next relapse is just around the corner that the outlook becomes bleak again.

Maintaining an optimistic view when faced with a setback of this kind is perfectly reasonable and once again will help our long-term progress. Viewing the setback as a small part of the entire journey can be helpful. So rather than focusing on any current difficulties in isolation, view them as existing after a long period of stability and with another long period of stability to come in the future, rather like a single obstacle on a long, straight, clear road.

Remaining optimistic after setbacks is an important part of the overall journey; pessimism can be quite damaging

It could be useful to actually draw this image on paper, with signposts along the way marking your progress in the past and your directions for the future.

We will look at the reasons for these setbacks in a moment, but whether a trigger has been identified or not, many choose to 'tighten up' their lifestyle as a reaction to a relapse or new symptom. This is empowering. You might like to think of this as preventing further deterioration and it could look like adding a few more raw vegetables to your diet, perhaps in the form of a daily juice, exercising more, or increasing the amount of meditation, yoga or other stress-reduction techniques in your life.

For some people who have avoided pharmaceutical options up to this point, a setback can be a chance to reconsider that decision, and they may choose to add in one of the pharmaceutical treatments for a time with a view to doing 'whatever it takes' to overcome the illness. How long after the previous relapse the setback occurs and how severe the symptoms are will probably be contributing factors in the decision. Accessing counselling, keeping a journal and temporarily reducing hours at work are all reasonable steps people take to regain a sense of control after experiencing a setback.

But why does it sometimes happen? If we have stabilised the illness, why do we sometimes get flare-ups after many years of stability?

Lifestyle treatment only works when you follow it

The first and most obvious answer is that sometimes, for many different reasons, people lapse on the OMS Program. Sometimes the lapse might be in one aspect, such as diet, with you deciding to eat certain foods that are not recommended. This could be for convenience, or just that it is what everyone else around you is doing. It often begins with one food item, and over time stretches to more and more types of food until your diet no longer resembles the Program recommendations at all.

Sun exposure and, for some, even vitamin D intake, are notoriously hard to keep up during winter, making this another aspect of the Program that some people find hard to follow. One former retreat participant stored his vitamins away in a cupboard instead of leaving them out on the bench where he could see them. As a result he forgot to take them. When he experienced a relapse after many years of stability he was actually happy to find that his vitamin D was deficient as it provided a clear reason for the setback. Correcting a vitamin D deficiency is easy with a one-off megadose or injection. After that it's just a case of keeping a careful eye on your weekly supplements or time in the sun.

Setbacks should initially prompt a review of how well you are adhering to the OMS Program

The aim of the Program is ultimately for the lifestyle to become automatic, so that we don't feel we are having to 'fit it in' to our lives. But in reality some of us are better at doing that than others, and if everyone around us is living a different way it's important to make sure we are really doing all the things we intend to be doing to remain well.

So, undoubtedly, some of us over time do drift away from the Program in one or more aspects, almost unconsciously. The relapse, when it comes, can be a timely reminder to tighten up our lifestyle measures or keep a closer eye on how we are implementing the Program recommendations.

Stress as a trigger

Many unexpected setbacks may seem random but, in fact, there is a clear correlation between the food that we eat, the vitamins that we take, the exercise and meditation that we do and the way MS shows up in our bodies. Since adopting these healthy habits helps our health stabilise, it is no surprise that reintroducing less healthy habits may cause a destabilisation. Nothing unpredictable about that!

Sometimes, though, relapses can occur even when we are doing everything we can and appear to have stabilised the illness. It's hard to know for certain why this is. All of us following the OMS Program are in some ways still pioneers; we rely on people's lived experience to know why potholes appear for some people but not for others. That said, stress appears to be a major contributing factor and setbacks are widely reported to follow stressful events, just like in the active stages of the illness. Stress is a plausible explanation, given its negative impact on the immune system.

Life, as we know, can be unpredictable. While we can influence the way that our bodies react to external events, we can't always influence the events themselves. For those of us who have reached stability on the OMS Program, we are mostly able to navigate the normal ups and downs and regular stresses of life, difficult periods at work, minor relationship troubles and financial worries. We probably have a well-developed meditation or stress-reduction routine that provides a certain amount of buffering from the impact of day-to-day stress.

Meditation and other forms of stress reduction are not foolproof; overwhelming stress can trigger a relapse despite using these techniques

Some major life events, however, are known to be the greatest causes of negative stress for everyone, with or without MS: the death of a loved one, divorce, redundancy and serious illness or injury. Sometimes, one or more of these events appear to trigger a setback even after many years of stability. My own story seems to fit into this category.

A personal perspective

My journey with MS began with a late-night phone call from the other side of the world sharing the devastating news that my father had broken his neck in a fall and was in a coma, not expected to survive. A few days later, sitting on a plane from Australia to the United Kingdom to attend his funeral, I noticed a sensation on my thighs that felt like sunburn even though I hadn't been in the sun. By the time the plane touched down in Brisbane two weeks later, both my legs had gone numb. I was 39 years old, happily married with three primary-school-aged children and a part-time job that I quite liked. The numbness in my legs spread to other parts of my body, fatigue set in and an MS diagnosis was made quickly, making sense of the mild sensory symptoms I'd noticed over the years. The disease became quite active from this point, with another relapse affecting my arms and upper body just a few months later. I was terrified and prepared to change my life in order to get better.

My route to recovery included embracing every aspect of the OMS Program, quitting my job to focus fully on my health for a while, attending an OMS retreat, eating a lot of raw vegetables and juices, seeking counselling for chronic anxiety, taking up running and meditating daily. I was fairly fanatical about the whole thing and incredibly determined. And I was rewarded with a lessening of symptoms and relapses that became milder and more spread out until after a couple of years they stopped altogether. I chose not to take pharmaceutical drugs but to stick to lifestyle modification to begin with, telling myself that I would reconsider if I had a major relapse.

Almost three years into the OMS Program I had my first stable MRI results, showing no active lesions and no new disease activity in a twelve-month period. From that point on I saw myself as recovering, subtly shifting my focus to one of maintaining good health rather than striving to achieve it. The running that I had taken up purely as a form of exercise became a hobby, eventually leading to my first half marathon. The meditation that I'd started for stress reduction took on a spiritual element as well. I started a new career as an instrumental music teacher, something I'd always wanted to do, and began writing songs again, recording two folk albums. My life was exciting, healthy and fulfilling and I got to the point of feeling that I would never have another relapse. It just didn't feel physically possible any more.

All was well for many years and then one night I got a phone call, much like the one I'd had before. This time it was my father-in-law who'd had a massive stroke and was not expected to survive. My husband was over in Scotland for his mum's funeral and this had happened quite unexpectedly to his dad just a few days afterwards.

The shock of that phone call went right through my body; it felt like something had broken. I was surprised by the intensity of my reaction, not realising at the time that I was reliving the trauma of receiving the news of my own dad's death nine years earlier. I was even standing in the same place in my house when I took the call, leaning against the dresser in my bedroom.

And just as my body had reacted the first time with an MS relapse, so the same thing happened again, even after seven years of stability and good health. It was four weeks before I felt the effect; I remember standing at the sink to wash up and finding that one hand felt like it had been plunged into icy water while the other felt quite warm. I soon discovered that one side of my body was affected in this way, with an abnormal reaction to water temperature whether in the shower, swimming pool or at the washing-up sink. I took a course of oral steroids, something I'd never actually done before for a relapse, and had an MRI scan that confirmed just one active lesion exactly where it would have been predicted from the symptoms. There were no other new lesions since my last scan, and two months later the disturbing symptoms were gone.

My initial reaction was to hide from the reality of the setback. I told almost no one yet I thought about it constantly and could see my mind inventing a very bleak future for myself quite different from the one that I'd been imagining in recent years. Breaking my silence was certainly helpful and allowed me to deal with my emotions. I booked in to see the therapist who had counselled me after diagnosis and turned to my usual support networks for help.

All was stable until the following year when, after another stressful life event, I once again noticed some new sensory symptoms. Surprisingly, when I had these checked out on MRI nothing showed up. Nevertheless, I had a strong sense that MS was the likely cause, a feeling my neurologist shared, so I looked at my lifestyle to see whether I could identify anything further that needed changing. The only tangible difference was my return to drinking alcohol after stopping for the first six years of my recovery. On reflection I decided that this was not helping my response to stress and even though moderate alcohol consumption is acceptable under the OMS Program, I opted to remain sober. I felt much better for it and have even wondered whether that was why I 'needed' to experience these symptoms. Counselling, journal writing and increased meditation all helped me to regain a sense of equilibrium.

On an emotional level I certainly overreacted to these setbacks, each time returning to the same place of dread that I'd been in on diagnosis. In reality, a couple of sensory episodes in nine years is a pretty good outcome, but it took some time for me to see it like that. Along the way I had to process feelings of guilt and shame and overcome the belief that I was a fraud and had let everyone down.

A role model of good health

Many people who have done very well following the OMS Program become role models for others in their communities: family members, friends, colleagues and sometimes even the general public. It can be heartening to know that others in the community look up to you as a beacon of hope. Many people choose, as I did, to tell their stories quite publicly, helping to spread the word that overcoming MS is possible. As we know, there are no guarantees, just the knowledge that good health is far more likely if you are following the Program. Still, having gone public with our story there is a sense for many of us that we are required to remain well, that our good health is as important to other people as it is to us.

This is not the case. In fact, while compassionate about my own plight, most people actually felt the setbacks made my recovery journey more real: 'Your story's actually better now; this makes it even more believable,' as one person put it. From others I had the sense that it made me more human, and therefore my achievements seemed more within reach to a lot of people. Whatever others' responses are, the fact is that your journey is yours alone and your first and only real obligation is to yourself.

There's no need for blame

It's easy to fall into 'what-ifs' when faced with a setback. People can ask, *What if I'd taken medication? What if I hadn't been doing such a demanding job?* But the problem with what-ifs is that they imply blame. What people are really saying is that perhaps you should have acted differently to avoid the relapse, it is your fault that this happened. But we cannot predict what is going to happen and the OMS Program is not a cure for the illness. There may still be some things that continue to affect us with MS but following the Program gives us the best chance of avoiding them.

Ground covered

One of the biggest causes of anxiety for people with MS is the unpredictable nature of the illness. Relapses or deterioration can occur at any time, affecting any part of the body's function, and this in turn makes it hard to plan or imagine a happy, rewarding future.

Adopting the OMS Program gives people with MS the best possible chance of ongoing good health and for many people this leads to permanent stability. However, some people experience an unexpected setback even after many years. This can be hard to deal with and often brings back many of the negative emotions that were present in the first few years after diagnosis.

Drifting away from the Program and traumatic or stressful events appear to be triggers for such setbacks but whatever the reason, the route back to good health is the same. The lifestyle that made you well in the first place is the one that can help you stabilise after an unexpected setback and return you to ongoing good health.

19

The road ahead

Professor George Jelinek

I started the OMS Program from an extremely
sceptical place, not believing that it would stop the
downward slope I was on; within three months . . .
I no longer needed a cane, and now I work out regularly and feel stronger than I have in many years.

Paula Cogan Myers, Mifflinburg, USA, OMSer

So we have learned about the lay of the land from a US neurologist, and we have explored the OMS Program and how to follow
it, with positive examples set by a broad range of people who
have embraced the Program and seen their lives change. We've
read personal stories and a number of direct quotes from people
with MS internationally. We now have a pretty good idea what
a difference the Program is making to the lives of people with MS.
Now we come to the road ahead. Let's consider what lies before
us, what may be possible in the future and the whole notion of
recovery from MS.

You may not have heard the word 'recovery' used by any of
your healthcare team. Hopefully, you will have heard it from
Overcoming Multiple Sclerosis. As an organisation founded on the
premise that it is possible not only to stabilise MS but to overcome
it, we are here to tell you that overcoming MS is possible. We have,
however, never disseminated the idea that the OMS Program is
somehow a cure for MS. It is not. It is a whole-of-life change

based on the best available science that uses every tool available to us as people with MS to reduce our risk of progression once diagnosed, and to reduce the risk of our loved ones developing the illness. The contributors of chapters, stories and quotes for this book, and many of the tens of thousands of people following the Program all over the world, attest that achieving these aims is possible. While many people with MS on the Program report that they have slowed the rate of deterioration, others also report that they have overcome the illness, that they have recovered and are now healthier than they were before diagnosis. But they are not cured. Their ongoing health depends on them continuing to embrace healthy lifestyle choices.

But before we go into what constitutes recovery, let's talk about the road ahead, the signposts on the way, and how a good outcome from MS might evolve for you.

Integrating the OMS Program into life

The recommendations for following the OMS Program are actually pretty simple, and of course very much open to individual variation and interpretation to fit into our own unique lives, as outlined in Part 2 of this book. But one can't just retreat from the world, become a hermit, and spend every waking moment focused on implementing the lifestyle recommendations. That isn't the point of the Program. The aim is actually to integrate this ultra-healthy lifestyle into one's daily life so that it becomes seamless. So that it requires no particular effort. So that it is actually enjoyable. And then one can engage fully with life, without much of the usual burden imposed by a progressive, disabling neurological illness, but equally without feeling that the price of this good health is itself a burden.

This takes time, and a gradual building of confidence and faith in oneself and the process. It is this faith that is the antidote to the anxiety and uncertainty that generally stalk people with MS. Anxiety that the next relapse or deterioration is just around the corner; uncertainty about the future and all the difficulties that it may hold. In a sense, the OMS Program is really a kind of 'set and forget' recipe for good health that doesn't require constant focus once it is established in one's life. As we have said many times, these very healthy lifestyle behaviours are habits, just like the old bad habits, except they are good. Once the habit of living well is ingrained, it is very easy to stick to, just like the old ones in fact. In the early days, fear may well drive the establishment and maintenance of the habit. But over time, the joy of living well and feeling great supersedes that.

So, as time passes by on the Program, for many people there is a gradual lessening of the initial anxiety that is replaced by a steadily building sense of calm and confidence. Confidence that once these lifestyle habits have been adopted and are ingrained, for most of us, the future will take care of itself. All the little things we do every day, more and more in a subconscious and routine way, cement in place the building blocks of a future of vitality and good health. This actually leaves us free to get on with life. In practice, what that looks like for many people on the Program is an open, engaged person developing healthy routines, moving in supportive social and work circles, and gradually being thought of by those around them as a particularly healthy individual with no particular health problems.

It sounds easy, but is it?

Of course, everyone's journey is different. For many people on the OMS Program over a number of years, this scenario is exactly what plays out: a healthy, happy life relatively free of the usual problems associated with MS. This is particularly so for those who come to the Program soon after diagnosis. For those who have already accumulated significant disability, the journey may be somewhat different. We don't pretend that it will always be easy or, for that matter, successful. One can imagine the amount of damage to sensitive structures in the brain and spinal cord that leads to significant disability. While our experience and feedback have been that there is often an improvement in disability with long-term adherence to the Program, and for some even complete or semi-complete reversal, for others the outcome may be continuing stability in the face of what was previously a steady decline.

Others still, despite adoption and adherence to the OMS Program over time, find that they nevertheless deteriorate. This is not a common outcome for those who report their stories back to us, but it does happen. The feedback we get from most of these people nevertheless is that the lifestyle changes are still worth it. Maintaining the Program actually does often provide many benefits even in the face of physical deterioration. Many report less fatigue, others that their quality of life is actually improved despite some physical decline, and others that long-term depression has lifted and their mood is brighter. That they are optimistic, involved and engaged with life despite their health difficulties.

Recovery

By far the stories we hear are more positive and more hopeful than that, though. Mostly, in our experience, people do not deteriorate on the OMS Program. Indeed, there are many stories of recovery, in line with the personal stories and some of the quotes we have seen in this book, representing just a handful of the people we know who are on the Program and who update us on their progress. But what constitutes recovery? Is it a word that should even be used in the same sentence as MS? Some healthcare professionals will start talking about 'false hope' when we talk about recovery. The notion of 'false hope', however, in this context is deeply flawed and comes from a very pessimistic view of the illness.

Talking about recovery after a diagnosis of MS is not 'false hope'

As our research from the STOP MS and HOLISM studies (referred to in *Overcoming Multiple Sclerosis* (2nd edition, 2016) or in PubMed or Google Scholar) keeps reminding us, many people with MS who are adopting healthy lifestyle behaviours are leading markedly different lives than have traditionally been associated with MS. For these people, the spectre of MS has essentially disappeared from their lives. Karen Law and I put a dozen of these stories into our book *Recovering from Multiple Sclerosis* (2013), and there are many more inspirational personal stories in this current book. On social media and the OMS website, one can read about the large number of people with MS who are now in good physical and mental health after adopting the OMS Program. Positive recovery stories are common, including of people being 'discharged' by their neurologists because they are too well to be followed up regularly and have not had new brain or spinal cord lesions over many years.

So 'false hope' in this situation is really 'false no hope'. People are being told that decline is inevitable, whereas we can see that the lives of a great number of people with MS actually get better. Not only do they not deteriorate, they improve. This is recovery. It is only reasonable to hope that you too can be one of these people. That is not 'false hope'; it is real hope. As the oncologist Carl Simonton once said, 'In the face of uncertainty, there is nothing wrong with hope.' More to the point, without hope there really is no way forward. Receiving the diagnosis of MS can be so shattering that without hope many of us just descend into depression. Becoming motivated, positive, hopeful and adopting a new, healthier and more engaged lifestyle are real antidotes to this descent. After all, at the time of diagnosis, most of us are well, even though we may still have the symptoms that led us to seek medical advice. Why waste this valuable time worrying about the future, when we are actually quite well? And of course, that future may never come to pass; the future may very well be bright.

Adopting an ultra-healthy lifestyle promotes recovery from many common chronic diseases; MS is no exception

Recovery is actually possible from a whole range of chronic diseases. And mostly, the formula for recovery is remarkably similar to the one presented here. An ultra-healthy diet, exercise, stress reduction and giving up bad habits like smoking and overeating will, for many people, deliver recovery from heart disease, high blood pressure and type 2 diabetes, and the list goes on. It is becoming clear as we do more and more research on lifestyle and MS that MS behaves in a fairly similar way to these other chronic Western diseases.

So what does a person who has recovered from heart disease look like? Well, a good example is Bill Clinton, former president of the United States. Bill was a junk food 'aholic'. If you watched some of his press briefings in the early days of his presidency, he'd often be out the front of a fast-food outlet eating his favourite fried chicken, doughnuts or burger. After cardiac bypass and stenting procedures, he decided he needed to change or he wouldn't live longer than his 58 years at the time. He enlisted the help of well-known cardiologist Dr Dean Ornish and over a number of years turned his condition around. He is now lean, healthy and, above all, still alive!

I have seen many people with MS in the same situation, coming to a residential workshop about lifestyle modification (retreat) in fairly poor health, overweight, eating badly, not exercising, depressed. After a week on retreat to kickstart their motivation, and then years of rigorous adherence to a healthier lifestyle, they end up looking, and indeed are, transformed. Many take up running, with some even completing marathons for the first time, years after a diagnosis of MS. While of course the field of medicine relies on solid scientific evidence about the potential benefit of such lifestyle changes, and of that there is plenty, there is nothing like seeing in the flesh such a profound change, or better still, being the person who changes. And that is possible for a great many people diagnosed with MS. There is simply no question about that.

Arriving at a healthier future

While everybody's response to modifying their lifestyle habits will be somewhat different, the research and our experience of the OMS community suggest that those who adhere more closely to the OMS Program recommendations do better in terms of the important health outcomes, including quality of life, fatigue and depression, but also relapses and disability. I have lost count of the number of people who have come back to a second or even third retreat saying that their initial enthusiasm ensured that they adhered to the guidelines very closely, only to find themselves 'falling off the wagon' over a period of years, and needing a refresher.

The universal theme from these people is that when they were really motivated and adhering rigorously they felt great, but that once that started waning they noticed small reminders of the illness returning, such as old symptoms that had disappeared, worsening fatigue, and so on, or frankly relapsing again and experiencing a new symptom like a deterioration in walking. After their refresher and a renewed commitment to healthier lifestyles, those who have kept in touch report noticing their vitality returning, their mood lifting and their endurance improving.

In general, the more rigorously one adopts the OMS Program, the better the likelihood of achieving results

Exercise is often a key part of this process, as Dr Stuart White reminds us in Chapter 5. The data show clearly that regular exercise is one of the more potent ways of improving fatigue. A vicious cycle can begin where one loses enthusiasm for exercise, feels more fatigued and lower in mood and less like exercising, and muscles start to lose power from lack of use, leading to further worsening of the whole spiral. Breaking that cycle and re-committing to regular exercise, in whatever form is possible and most suits the individual, can turn the whole thing around. And any exercise is better than none.

It should probably come as no surprise that the more we invest in our own health, the more we get back. It's what we would expect in most things we do. Similarly, setting our goals and aims high often translates into achieving more, again just as it does in other endeavours. I have had participants at retreats say that their aim is to slow down the deterioration; others have said that they want to return to full health and recover. It is amazing how often these become self-fulfilling prophecies. Or perhaps we shouldn't be amazed. Once we set a certain intention in our minds, both consciously and subconsciously we start to work towards that goal. Aim high. You might just get there.

What to expect

In terms of outlining what might be possible for you and what to expect over the decades after committing to an ultra-healthy life-style plan like the OMS Program, I thought it would probably be best and most authentic if I painted a picture of my own progress since diagnosis. I am sure others who have been on the Program for many years will have had different experiences. But I am equally sure that similarities will probably outweigh differences. We are all individuals with our own preconceptions, personalities and ways of doing things. But again, there are so many more similarities between people than differences I think, particularly when we are faced with one of the most life-altering diagnoses one can receive.

The first five years

Drawing on my own experience of these years, a number of themes come through. While these are personal, I suspect that there may be some universality about some of the emotions and signposts that arose for me during these years.

Over the first five years, anxiety and uncertainty, if not frank fear and despondency, were dominant feelings, particularly in the early times after diagnosis. Very fortunately, I had some wonderful guides and navigated that period in a way that enabled me to find enormous hope and optimism quite quickly. That centred around the discovery and implementation of information that impelled me to write the first edition of *Taking Control of Multiple Sclerosis* in 1999, becoming the first edition of *Overcoming Multiple Sclerosis* in 2010. The original research findings were refined a little over the years into what became known as the OMS Program. The sense of empowerment that I got from discovering how I could help myself is really what provided the impetus for my recovery. In Chapter 10 Dr Sam Gartland talks about having similar feelings

Doing something positive about the disease provides a great sense of control

in the early period after diagnosis. He is now ultra-fit and the healthiest he has ever been, working as a GP in New South Wales, Australia.

But it is perfectly natural to feel negative emotions early on after diagnosis. Some people fall back on denial as a way of dealing with these emotions, looking away from rather than facing the truth of one's possible future. Actually engaging fully with the reality of the diagnosis and its potential consequences is a key component of overcoming MS, at least in my view. Repressing those emotions rather than actually feeling and processing them is a recipe for depression and long-term ill health, just as repressing unwanted or unpleasant feelings is harmful in other circumstances. Allowing the difficult emotions to just be there, working through them and coming to some acceptance of one's own feelings about the uncertain future and potential loss are important steps to take before one can really start a positive shift out of the dark days.

The next step is to take on board doing something about the illness. The challenge of fashioning a new life, with new ways of eating and living, marks the start of an exciting journey. Not only does physical health generally improve, but mental health and quality of life do as well, because of the sense of mastery that we gradually develop, the belief that we have control of our futures. Having a sense of being the master of one's own future is a great source of energy and optimism. It's hard, however, for me to imagine how I could have done so well over the years without a true acceptance of the reality of the diagnosis before embarking on this path.

Setting goals over those initial months is a good idea, at least it was for me. My early goal was to be relapse-free for six months. and then two years, then five years. I started a diary setting out these goals and documenting how I was feeling as I travelled that road. It's great to go back and read that diary now and see the hope and the sense of excitement that I had, how a devastating diagnosis turned into a real adventure, full of highs and lows, and gradually a transformation of my life.

For some the disease is very active initially and it can be difficult to get any sense of control if there are continual relapses and
worsening symptoms. Feeling fatigued and physically ill a lot of
the time can be very difficult to live with, and can have a profound
effect on mood. For many people, this prompts an early decision
to begin treatment with one of the more potent disease-modifying
medications, accepting that while they may have a negative impact
on quality of life, the potential benefits may outweigh the risks
of a very active disease course. This may provide enough stability to give the lifestyle changes more chance of being effective,
given that they can take some years
to achieve maximal benefit. These are
personal decisions, made of course in
consultation with one's health advisers.
But committing to doing everything
possible, 'whatever it takes', is a key
strategy that we recommend.

*Taking one of the
'disease-modifying
therapies' is an
important part of
the 'whatever it
takes' approach for
many people*

I opted to take one of the available
medications at around seven months
after diagnosis when a new lesion
appeared on an MRI scan and I was
experiencing profound fatigue. With that help, I felt somewhat
more in control and was able to achieve some stability by the end
of my first year after diagnosis. Armed with that sense of greater
control, I found that at around three to four years, I had begun to
reset my bearings. I didn't even know that I was doing it, but the
mere act of finally really looking after myself meant that my priorities were starting to change. Relationships, family, social circle,
work—it all began changing. I found my life changing in ways
that I didn't imagine, and in some ways was not prepared for. But
I was fundamentally changing and went with the changes rather
than resisting them.

The first five to ten years
After getting to the five-year mark with no neurological disability,
a goal that I scarcely believed was possible when I started, I began

to notice a gradually developing sense of calm and stability in my internal life and feelings, although there was still a lot of turbulence in my external day-to-day life. I still felt some uncertainty and even anxiety about relapsing, but I had developed enough faith in myself and the process to be calm about it and let those emotions go. Much of the tumult of the first five years after diagnosis had passed by this stage. My friendships and relationships were in the process of reordering. I still had a sense of discomfort about that, and sometimes much more than discomfort, particularly about losing some long-standing relationships, but again I was letting those feelings go more and more and just allowing my life to proceed without too much sense of control or planning from me.

One particularly valuable tool over this time was mindfulness meditation. Learning to better let go of difficult thoughts and emotions was a really important part of the whole lifestyle package that I had adopted. I found meditation extremely important too for adapting to change, and not ruminating about things that I was leaving behind or moving away from. While some people say that they simply can't meditate, that their mind is too active, that they can't sit still long enough, these are the very people who most need to learn that skill. And it is a skill. Many people want results quickly, but it takes practice to develop the skill of meditation. It is a very powerful tool that works not only directly in a physiological way to improve health by counteracting the effects of stress, but also in deeper ways. One learns to cultivate a sense of comfort with difficult situations through continually practising not being distracted by troublesome thoughts and by learning to stay more in the present moment.

Regular mindfulness meditation is not just about dealing with stress; quite simply, it improves life

One particular cause for discomfort started to become more obvious during this time. My relationship with my work and career became less and less solid as I started to actively question whether what I was doing satisfied and fulfilled me. I gave up many of the leadership roles that I had held within my career in emergency medicine, and began to focus more on my passion, which was to help to spread the message to people with MS about what was possible. While it took me quite some years to finally walk away from my enormously stressful clinical career, the process started very soon after diagnosis as I learned to be comfortable with change.

I also began to question my decision to take disease-modifying drugs. For the first five years I had religiously taken a daily dose of Copaxone. Indeed, I don't recall ever missing a dose during this period. I remember getting quite nervous if there was ever any delay in its delivery to my local pharmacy. But over the next five years, I started to question whether the medication was actually doing anything for me over and above what the lifestyle changes were doing, given that the medication didn't really purport to keep people with MS well, just to reduce the number of relapses somewhat. And I was perfectly well. Increasingly I wondered whether I should have a trial period off the medication.

So over the course of a year or two, in discussion with my new neurologist, I reduced the frequency of the medication until I was finally off it altogether. While this did feel a little risky, the sense of autonomy and mastery that I gained was enormous. I no longer felt like a patient but simply a normal, very healthy man in his mid-fifties. And I was.

At around the same time, I stopped talking about 'my MS' or 'my illness' but rather referred to having been diagnosed with MS. This movement away from having the illness to having once been diagnosed with it was metaphorically very important. It wasn't that I was denying the diagnosis, or that I was in any way pretending or feeling that I was 'cured'. Rather, I started to sense that I was actually beginning to heal. And the healing was not only physical but much deeper. I was starting to feel much more comfortable in my own skin. Many longstanding emotional issues, particularly those

The language that we use about the illness is important; it doesn't have to be 'my' MS

around the death of my mother, began to dissipate. The sense of 'dis-ease' that I had come to realise was contributing to physical disease was losing its intensity. I didn't really feel like I had a disease anymore. I started to feel free of it and so decided that I no longer needed to 'own' it; it wasn't my disease anymore.

The second decade

To make it to the second decade from diagnosis in good health was something I had never really dared to believe was possible. But to make it through the second decade and into a third seemed like a miracle. And in a sense, it was, and is. To have done it has really cemented my conviction that overcoming MS is possible. Over the course of that second ten years since diagnosis, MS became a research focus and a passion, as I strove to promote the message about overcoming MS, and something that brought many, many friends into my life. It was no longer the painful, frightening, dark companion that I had thought it would be throughout my whole life. I was now able to believe that recovery from MS was possible, not just lessening the impact or managing symptoms or coping, but the genuine possibility of being free of any manifestation of the disease. This was how my life was turning out.

The constant spectre of MS hanging over my head, the sword about to fall at any moment, was gone. While it may have seemed that life had returned to how it had been pre-diagnosis, in fact that was not at all true. Life was very different, because I was fundamentally different. My passions, goals, desires, the whole inner and outer landscapes of my life were different. I had changed, and while it had been extremely challenging, overall I was glad that I had changed, MS or no MS. This is what the OMS Program advocates: change your life, for life! The process of overcoming MS can lead to a journey of personal transformation. It is not just about changing habits, or overcoming a disease. In fact, once we commit to a path like this, everything about life changes. Work, family, friendships, aspirations—everything. While at the beginning it felt like a giant hand had reached in and taken away my future, what really happened was that I rebuilt an entirely different future. Through the process of making all the lifestyle changes, through regular meditation, through re-evaluating everything about life. MS, the illness, had lost its direct relevance to the person I now was.

What my life looked like externally mirrored this internal change. By the latter part of the second decade after diagnosis, I was no longer working in emergency medicine; I was heading a research unit at Australia's most highly ranked university specifically studying lifestyle factors in MS and how they affect disease progression. My work and my life felt aligned at last with my inner landscape. What I did for a job was what I lived and breathed in my life and had developed as a result of all the choices I had made in response to the illness.

The long journey to recovery

Recovery is an interesting and multifaceted phenomenon. For me, it felt like my recovery was from much more than just an illness. Along the way, my ambition fell away, my desire for achievement and success gave way to finding fulfillment and satisfaction in my work and life. Lots of the demons that had plagued me as a young man were tamed along the way. My recovery was as much from overcoming them as overcoming MS. And I feel sure that I am not alone in this. Many people who have written personal stories for this book and many, many others who have contacted me over the years talk about similar journeys.

But as a well-trained, mainstream medical specialist, I am a realist. I fully acknowledge that my story will not be everybody's outcome or story. There will be some whose experience of MS is anything but positive. I deliberately focus on the positives, given how many voices you will hear talking about the negatives and how bad the future will be after a diagnosis of MS, including those of many of our own health advisers. That is not to say that I am unaware of the negatives. I watched my mother's life deteriorate into the most profoundly disturbing end of life I could have then imagined, and a relatively young life at that. I understand the cruelty of this disease if left unchecked. But nothing was known about the role of lifestyle factors in MS progression back in the 1960s and 70s. And there were no medications that could help.

That has all changed. There is a growing scientific evidence base behind the lifestyle changes and disease-modifying therapies we have outlined in this book. Slowing progression of the disease, stability, and outright recovery are all possible outcomes in the spectrum of the course of this illness after committing to lifestyle change. While there are of course no guarantees, for many, overcoming MS is possible. If you haven't already started on the OMS Program, today might be a good day to begin the journey.

Ground covered

There are numerous possible paths following a diagnosis of MS. Historically, most of these have been very negative. The advent of disease-modifying therapies has provided genuine medical treatments that can slow disease progression. The emerging science around adoption of an ultra-healthy lifestyle program adds considerably to this optimism.

For many people with MS, overcoming MS has become a realistic proposition. A large number are now living very positive lives, free from the usual problems associated with this illness. Adopting the OMS Program can lead to much deeper, personal changes and life can be transformed for many people with MS. It is not a quick fix, but every small step towards a healthier lifestyle will be rewarded in what can realistically be a healthy, fulfilling future.

Index

exercise
5 'Cs' 101
aerobic, regular 37, 91, 94, 102
aids to 103
amount of 92
anaerobic 91
barriers to 97–9
being lax about 33
benefits of 88, 95, 164, 165, 188, 208, 232
best exercise 91
cardiovascular 164
changing 100
checking 100
committing to 99
consistency 100
cooling down before 102
daily record of 104
depression and 37, 89, 232
endorphins 232
enough, getting 32
fatigue and 38, 89, 232, 342
form, importance of 164–5
functional 164
goal-setting 100, 165
gyms, cost of 98
hydrotherapy 103
illness, preventing 89
importance of 37, 342
inflammation 90
lack of 90
medicine, as 208
mental and psychological wellbeing 89
MS and 87
nervous system, effects of 89
new lifestyle, in 88
new routines for 254
outdoor physical activities 165, 254
overcoming barriers to 95
PMS, for people with 163–5
pump classes 310
reasons for 88
regular 99, 188, 232, 254, 342
right sort, getting 37
socialising and 100
spiritual benefits 89
strength training 94
stretching exercises 91
swimming 103
temperature and 101–2

too much 92
types of 94, 102
water, in 103
wellness, maintaining 89
why exercise works 90
exercise physiologist 208
Expanded Disability Status Score (EDSS) 10, 11, 12

falls
exercise, effect of 38, 98
fear of falling 98
'false hope', notion of 339–40
family
starting a family 289–91
family members
altering risk of 185
disclosure of diagnosis to 279–82
emotions of 281
lifestyle modifications by 189–90
preventing MS in 183
risk of developing MS 15, 184
sun exposure 189
support of 207, 313, 315
farmers' markets 312
fast foods 33
fathers
MS medication taken by 299
fatigue
exercise, effect of 38, 89, 232, 342
lessening impact of 49
low vitamin D 70, 73
medications for 23
OMS Program helping to prevent 271
OMS Program recommendations, adhering to 341
sun exposure and 75
symptom, as 13, 32, 38
work, from 271
fats
blood profile, in 48
'essential fatty acids' 54
managing, in diet 54
omega-3 fatty acids see omega-3 fatty acids
role of 55
saturated see saturated fats
seafood, in 53
substitutes 56
texture of food, changing 55